The Essential Guide TO

Caring for Aging Parents

by Dr. Linda Rhodes

ALPHA BOOKS

Published by Penguin Group (USA) Inc.

Penguin Group (USA) Inc., 375 Hudson Street, New York, New York 10014, USA • Penguin Group (Canada), 90 Eglinton Avenue East, Suite 700, Toronto, Ontario M4P 2Y3, Canada (a division of Pearson Penguin Canada Inc.) • Penguin Books Ltd., 80 Strand, London WC2R 0RL, England • Penguin Ireland, 25 St. Stephen's Green, Dublin 2, Ireland (a division of Penguin Books Ltd.) • Penguin Group (Australia), 250 Camberwell Road, Camberwell, Victoria 3124, Australia (a division of Pearson Australia Group Pty. Ltd.) • Penguin Books India Pvt. Ltd., 11 Community Centre, Panchsheel Park, New Delhi—110 017, India • Penguin Group (NZ), 67 Apollo Drive, Rosedale, North Shore, Auckland 1311, New Zealand (a division of Pearson New Zealand Ltd.) • Penguin Books (South Africa) (Pty.) Ltd., 24 Sturdee Avenue, Rosebank, Johannesburg 2196, South Africa • Penguin Books Ltd., Registered Offices: 80 Strand, London WC2R 0RL, England

International Standard Book Number: 978-1-61564-191-8
Library of Congress Catalog Card Number: 2011945185

14   13   12   8   7   6   5   4   3   2   1

Interpretation of the printing code: The rightmost number of the first series of numbers is the year of the book's printing; the rightmost number of the second series of numbers is the number of the book's printing. For example, a printing code of 12-1 shows that the first printing occurred in 2012.

Printed in the United States of America

Note: This publication contains the opinions and ideas of its author. It is intended to provide helpful and informative material on the subject matter covered. It is sold with the understanding that the author and publisher are not engaged in rendering professional services in the book. If the reader requires person̶ ̶ ̶ ̶ ̶ ̶ ̶ ̶ ̶ ̶ ̶ ̶, a competent professional should be consulted.

̶ ̶nsibility for any liability, loss, or risk, ̶ ̶ ̶ ̶ ̶ ̶ ̶ ̶directly or indirectly, of the use and

̶ ̶ ̶ ̶ ̶ ̶ ̶r bulk purchases for sales promotions, ̶ ̶ ̶ ̶ook excerpts, can also be created to

̶ ̶ ̶ ̶ ̶et, New York, NY 10014.

̶ ̶ ̶ta Hansing Editorial Services, Inc.
̶ ̶ ̶**igner:** Rebecca Batchelor
̶ ̶becca Batchelor, William Thomas
̶ ̶ ̶**er:** Celia McCoy
̶ ̶ ̶: Ayanna Lacey
̶ ̶ ̶**ader:** Laura Caddell

PEARSON

Dedication

To my sister, Mary Joyce (Jodi) Gorman, my best friend and unwavering partner in caring for Mom and Dad.

Contents

Appendixes

Introduction

Caregiving is saintly, but it shouldn't lead to martyrdom. Over the last 10 years, I've received countless questions from readers of my newspaper column, "Our Parents, Ourselves," on what to do and how to care for older parents. Some questions portray a family facing a crisis, while others grapple with elder care issues over the long haul. Whatever the question or the nature of their circumstance, families want quick, knowledgeable, common-sense answers that can help them *do right* by their loved ones.

But beyond answers on what to do, I've come to appreciate the dynamics among family members as they care for their older loved ones. Some of the more frequent questions I receive focus on how to better communicate with siblings and parents, how to work through differences of opinion on what's best for Mom or Dad, and how to handle the stress of caregiving.

I've written this book to address not only the "what and how" surrounding elder care, but also what's at the heart of the matter: families.

Families are the backbone of elder care; without them, millions of older relatives would age under dire and lonely circumstances. Yet families are stretched so thin today: they are juggling careers while caring for two and three generations, living long distance, coping with the challenges of blended families, and managing geriatric health-care demands they never imagined. It frays nerves and makes communicating wearing and reaching consensus daunting.

This book offers a unique blend of answers on the "what and how" of caregiving, along with tools and tips to help you solve problems, resolve differences, and bring organization and peace of mind to your caregiving.

Just remember to take care of yourself while you care for others. And thank you for trusting me to accompany you on your caregiving journey.

May you and those you love age well.

How to Use This Book

The book is written in five parts that walk you through various aspects of caregiving, each providing the essential tools and knowledge to confidently and compassionately care for your parents. What makes this book unique is my companion website to the book that hyperlinks the entire Resource Directory and caregiving videos, and provides caregiver forms and worksheets referenced in the book that you can share with family members and physicians. All are available for free on my website, at www. lindarhodescaregiving.com. Here's a quick rundown of each part:

Part 1, Problem Solving Amid Confusion, shows you how to observe and identify signs and symptoms in your parents, tells you what a geriatric assessment can do, and teaches you how to talk about health issues with your parent. Learn how to clearly define a problem, identify caregiving tasks, and get other family members to pitch in. Gain insights on your parent's perspective and learn why you must take care of yourself.

Part 2, The Elder Care Landscape: Know More, Act Confidently, prepares you to scope out the best living options, learn how to access reports on their quality, track down public benefits and caregiving services, and get a heads-up on the basic legal questions every caregiver needs to know.

Part 3, Managing Medical Life, shows you how to act as your parent's advocate in the doctor's office, in the hospital, in the emergency department, and through the insurance maze. Find out what questions to ask and what information to have at your fingertips. And discover what your loved one needs during end-of-life care and when to reach out to hospice.

Part 4, Family Dynamics in the Swirl of Caregiving, recognizes that caregiving is intertwined with family and that emotions can run high because the stakes are high. In this part, you gain a better understanding of the generational differences between baby boomers and their parents, learn to refocus your relationship with your siblings, determine your caregiving style, and find out how to set realistic expectations.

Part 5, Communicating in Sync, tackles a skill that is especially useful for families grappling with caregiving issues. In this part, you discover your communication style and its effect in working with your parents and siblings. You also see how your money style influences the choices you and your parent make on elder care and how it can lead to conflict. This part also helps you learn how to communicate with a loved one struggling with Alzheimer's disease and other forms of dementia.

Essential Extras

Throughout the book, you'll find added information to enhance what's being discussed. You'll find this in three types of sidebars:

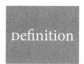

Definitions of important caregiving words or phrases.

Warnings and helpful hints on what to do for added protection.

Helpful tools and savvy tips to make your caregiving easier, including invaluable resources, help lines, and contacts.

You'll also see a fourth, name-changing sidebar that presents quotes, interesting facts, or other extended background information you should know.

Acknowledgments

Special thanks go to my technical reviewer and colleague during my tenure as Secretary of Aging, Bob Hussar, former Chief of the Division of Consumer Protection for the Pennsylvania Department of Aging. Bob's career spanned more than 30 years in state government, overseeing all the Department of Aging's development of regulations and devising standards and regulations of the Pennsylvania's adult protective services program. To Pat Shull, RN, Chief Executive Officer; Kimberly A. Marnien, CTRF, Director of Family Services; and Wendy Walsh, RN, Director of Staff Education at Adult Care of Chester County, thank you for sharing your insights on the needs of families who manage with sacrifice and love to maintain their loved ones at home because of what you do. I'm also grateful to Jenni Ellingson, of Public Works, LLC, who kept the ball moving by assisting with organizing my material for chapter development. Thanks also go to Brook Farling, Senior Acquisitions Editor of Alpha Books, who steered this book and this writer to the finish line, and to Ginny Munroe, for her words of encouragement and her adept editing of my words.

I am especially appreciative of my readers of the *Patriot–News* who keep me grounded by sharing their real-life stories and questions. They are my inspiration to keep on writing. And thanks, Mom and Dad, for all the experience you've given me in caring for you, as you did for me. The strength and dignity that each of you brings to whatever life throws at you is the stuff of quiet heroes. And to my husband, Eric, thanks for allowing me to be missing in action even as you never missed supporting me. And Matt and Brennan, my son and daughter, thanks for running errands, bringing me lunch, and cheering me on. Now you have an owner's manual on caring for your mom.

Special Thanks to the Technical Reviewer

The Essential Guide to Caring for Aging Parents was reviewed by an expert who double-checked the accuracy of what you'll learn here, to help us ensure that this book gives you the essentials on caring for aging parents. Special thanks are extended to Bob Hussar.

Trademarks

All terms mentioned in this book that are known to be or are suspected of being trademarks or service marks have been appropriately capitalized. Alpha Books and Penguin Group (USA) Inc. cannot attest to the accuracy of this information. Use of a term in this book should not be regarded as affecting the validity of any trademark or service mark.

Part 1

Problem Solving Amid Confusion

Whether caregiving enters your life in bits and pieces or in one fell swoop with a crisis or a life-changing diagnosis, you'll be confronted with problems—lots of problems that can generate a great deal of confusion.

Solving problems when you're not sure what's wrong, when Mom and Dad are at a loss or in denial, when family members disagree, and when everyone's feeling stressed rarely leads to good solutions. Certainly, it won't lead to the kinds of solutions that you or your parent can live with or that serve everyone's best interest.

To get a head start, learn to observe signs and symptoms during visits with your parents that point to issues that require your attention. Then try to appreciate your parent's viewpoint when it comes to addressing those topics. Find out how to define problems in a clear and focused way so that you can tackle them efficiently with the least amount of conflict. Discover tools and tips for organizing your caregiving that involve both your parent and other family members who have a stake in Mom or Dad's care.

No matter how well you and your parent handle caregiving, it will be stressful. It's why I've dedicated an entire chapter in Part 1 to helping you identify your own level of stress, the emotions that trigger it, and strategies to relieve it every day.

The act of caregiving is saintly, but it doesn't require martyrdom.

chapter 1

What's Really Wrong with My Parent?

> Telltale signs that should catch your attention
>
> Watching out for age-related conditions
>
> Why you'll want a geriatrician and geriatric assessment
>
> Delving into medical conditions

It's usually the little things that catch our attention. Despite our attempts to shrug them off and continue with our busy lives, we reach the point when we can no longer ignore them. Mom's outfits don't match, despite her celebrated history of color-coordinating her blouses, skirts, shoes, and purses. And *no* jewelry? She's never without her earrings. Phone conversations with Dad seem a little disjointed, and he hasn't been watching his beloved sports shows. Bills aren't getting paid. And Mom, who loves an outing at the mall, complains that walking around is getting too much for her.

Signs of dementia? Could shortness of breath be causing Mom to shorten her walks? Is a heart problem lurking? Or are these simply signs of normal aging? Time to find out how to dig a little further and take action when needed.

Signs That Something Is Amiss

Let's take a moment to understand two kinds of aging: primary and secondary. We owe primary aging to our genes. In this case, we're essentially along for the ride as our DNA plays out "hereditary units" passed from parent to offspring. Primary aging explains why some men age with a full head of hair and some families clock 90 years without much of a hitch. But no matter how great those inherited genes are, your parents will experience a decline in what's known as *trophic factors*.

definition

Trophic comes from Greek, meaning to "feed or nourish." **Trophic factors** such as hormones and proteins nourish the growth, survival, and function of cells and neurons that help our bodies function.

Essentially, hormonal substances that our bodies produce—such as estrogen, testosterone, and human growth factors—decline as we age. When we start producing less of them, the classic signs of aging emerge: less height, hair, hair color, smooth skin, bone mass, and muscle fiber. Senses become less effective, resulting in hearing and vision loss. One of the more damaging trophic factors is a lessening of the immune system's ability to fight off infections such as pneumonia and the flu. It all sounds pretty familiar. It's what most people view as normal aging.

When it comes to secondary aging, your parents don't have to take a back seat to genetic coding. Moderate exercise, a healthy diet, and no smoking can prevent clogged arteries, keep lungs pumping at capacity, and strengthen muscles and bones. Engaging in volunteer activities, having a social life, and playing "brain fitness" games can keep the mind sharp and even stave off dementia.

Of course, the hard part is knowing what's normal and what's not, and what can be prevented and what should be treated. Over the years, I've developed a checklist of what to look for as signs that something could be amiss. I really don't run around with a clipboard when I'm visiting my parents, but I keep an eye out for signs of potential trouble ahead.

Here's what to investigate:

- **Explore around the house.** Are household bills piling up and is mail left unopened? This could be a sign that the simple tasks of writing bills, balancing a checkbook, and keeping track of due dates are becoming overwhelming. Do you see scorched pots and pans? Is the house more unkempt than usual? All these signs could flag a decrease in thinking skills, decreased vision, and/or an inability to physically handle household chores.

- **Check out the refrigerator.** Is it well stocked with fresh produce and meats, or do you see signs of a poor diet and moldy, expired food products? When you take your parents out to eat, are they eating a lot less and showing little interest in food? Do they appear to have lost weight? Are they drinking water throughout the day? Look for signs that your parents are becoming malnourished and/or dehydrated. Poor diet can exacerbate chronic diseases, lead to a weakened immune system, and increase the risk of dementia. Lack of appetite could also be a sign of depression.

- **Ask about their social life.** When was the last time they visited with friends? Went out to eat? Went to church? Did the things they loved doing? If you find them reluctant to leave the house, this could be a sign that they're having a hard time driving, moving about, seeing, or hearing. They may even be having a bladder problem, so they'd rather stay home than risk embarrassment. This could lead to loneliness and depression. Find out what's causing your parents to disengage.

- **Let them take you for a drive and go for a walk.** If your parents are still driving, you might do well to ride with them and let them take the steering wheel so you can assess their driving skills. You should especially do this if you see dents or scratches on the car, if either of them has talked about "near misses," or if a parent has received recent speeding or traffic tickets. In terms of walking, take a drive to the mall and see if they exhibit any shortness of breath, or watch them go up the stairs at home. If they need to take a break, explore why. You could see signs of a heart condition.

- **Check out their medications.** Are expired pill bottles mixed in with current ones? Are the pills organized to prevent them from taking the wrong dose or too many pills? Are they taking more than five medications? Do they have a list of the current medications they take, and do they bring it with them to every doctor's appointment? Can they explain to you what they take, for what, and at what time of day? Do they have a system for taking their medications, and can they show it to you? Up to 20 percent of hospital admissions among the elderly are due to an adverse drug event (ADE), and most of those could have been prevented.

- **Turn your phone call into a checkup.** Even when you're not visiting your parents, you can make your daily or weekly chat into a checkup without being annoying. Listen for repeated stories during your conversation or forgotten facts that they would rarely ever forget, such as grasping for names of family and close friends or getting dates mixed up. Weave into your conversation questions like these: What did they have for breakfast, lunch, or dinner? What happened during the last episode of their favorite television show? Find a way to ask today's date. You are looking for signs of confusion that could be related to a host of problems: dehydration, side effects of medication, high or low blood pressure, hypoglycemia (a sign of diabetic shock or, during a heat wave, a sign of a heat stroke). If you notice these types of behaviors repeatedly, it could be a sign of dementia.

So now you have a list of the little things to put on your radar screen. If they happen frequently (three times or more) and you're seeing a pattern, you need to dig deeper to find the underlying cause.

Alert

Being observant is always good, but don't be too quick to jump to conclusions at the first sign of possible trouble. Reactions to medications cause a wide range of side effects, some of which mimic dementia. And a simple build-up of earwax can cause people to lose their balance and fall.

Aging's Big Four

Aging is anything but static. It's a dynamic process and, just as dominoes fall in rapid succession, it doesn't take much for one problem to lead to another. The older you are, the more fragile your physiological state. You need a true understanding of how a geriatric body reacts to medicines, nutrition, surgeries, and so on. But just about all older people and their loved ones worry about four major health conditions: cancer, strokes, heart attacks, and Alzheimer's disease. It's a quadrangle of woe—yet with early intervention, a watchful eye, and aggressive treatment, many people can continue to live productive lives.

So let's get everyone's fears out in the open and go through the basics of each condition so you can focus on what to look for and what to do.

Heart Attacks

I can still see my dad's cardiologist pointing to an x-ray of his clogged artery and announcing, "This is the one we call the widow maker. It's 90 percent clogged." His physician was referring to my father's left coronary artery. Lucky for my dad, my sister saw him experiencing shortness of breath while he was going up the stairs. She's a nurse and promptly hauled him off to his primary doctor, who scheduled a series of tests. Fifteen years later, his stent (a meshlike device that holds open a narrowed coronary artery) is working just fine, at 91 years of age.

Four main conditions lead to heart attacks: high blood pressure, cholesterol, angina, and congestive heart failure. The following sections provide a brief recap of each of these.

High Blood Pressure

The continuous, high-pressured rush of blood coursing through arteries wears down their hoselike walls until a leak or tear is possible. Being overweight and eating a diet high in salt are the leading causes of high blood pressure. But your parent may not experience any symptoms of high blood pressure, which explains why this condition is known as a "silent killer." Some people with high blood pressure may experience a headache or dizziness, but the best way of knowing whether your parent has a problem is to have his or her blood pressure read.

Tip
A blood pressure reading consists of two numbers. The upper number measures the pressure in the arteries when the heart beats (systolic pressure); the lower number measures the pressure in the arteries between beats (diastolic pressure). According to the Mayo Clinic, a normal reading is around 120/80. Those with stage one hypertension have a blood pressure that reads 140 to 159 systolic pressure over 90 to 99 diastolic pressure. People with severe hypertension, at stage two, show a reading of 160/100 and higher.

If high blood pressure has already been a serious condition for your parent, buy an automated blood pressure cuff so that Mom or Dad can take a reading every day. If needed, your parent's doctor could prescribe a remote blood pressure device that reads blood pressure and transmits it over the phone to a medical office that will monitor the readings. Medications may also help reduce blood pressure, as can lifestyle and dietary changes.

Cholesterol

Blood vessels are small, and the best way for them to function is to stay clear so blood can easily flow to and from the heart. Cholesterol is a fatty, sticky substance that clogs those vessels, and too much blockage (athero-sclerosis) prevents adequate blood from flowing to the heart. Smoking, high blood pressure, diabetes, and a diet high in fats contribute to high levels of cholesterol.

Two kinds of cholesterol exist. The "good" kind, known as high-density lipoprotein (HDL), is produced naturally by the body and carries choles-terol away from the artery wall. "Bad" cholesterol, referred to as low-density lipoprotein (LDL), clogs the arteries and sets you up for a heart attack. Reducing animal fat in your parent's diet is key to bringing down LDL levels. Medications can also help. Given your parent's current cholesterol levels, ask the doctor how often your mom or dad should have it checked.

Angina

Temporary chest pains and a sensation of pressure around the heart are classic signs of angina. It's the heart signaling that it isn't receiving enough oxygen. Other symptoms are indigestion; shortness of breath; and an odd ache around the neck that spreads to the jaw, throat, shoulder, back, or arms. If your parent experiences any of these, he or she needs to see a doctor right away. This isn't one of those little things we talked about earlier.

Chances are, your parent will be given a number of tests—such as an EKG (electrocardiogram), stress tests, scans, and echocardiograms—to determine what's really going on. Another possible test is catheterization, a procedure in which thin tubing is inserted into a vein or artery and x-ray and dyes are then used to determine where and how much blockage lies within blood vessels. A wide range of procedures can correct the blockage, ranging from medications, to stents, to angioplasty (widening the vessel with a tiny balloon), to open-heart bypass surgery.

Congestive Heart Failure

In the case of congestive heart failure (CHF), your mom or dad's heart muscle is actually damaged and slowing the heart's blood flow. As a result, blood backs up into either the lungs or the veins, causing fluid congestion in the tissues. People with CHF can gain 2 to 4 pounds of fluid buildup overnight, which you'll see in swollen ankles, legs, or arms. Tiredness, a hacking cough, shortness of breath, and a sensation of suffocating are all signs of CHF. The term *failure* can be pretty frightening, but it's not necessarily a death sentence. CHF can be managed by medications and a heart-healthy diet.

> **Tip**
>
> The American Heart Association provides a treasure trove of information on heart disease, including how to manage it, symptoms to watch for, reviews on the latest research, and animated videos to explain heart disease and various procedures to address it. They even have a special section just for caregivers. Visit the AHA at www.heart.org or call 1-800-242-8721.

Brain Attacks

Most of us know these as strokes, but the medical community now refers to them as brain attacks, which actually makes more sense. Just as a heart attack results in less blood and oxygen reaching the heart, the brain suffers the same loss in a stroke. A clogged artery or a vessel tear may leak blood before or after blood reaches the brain. How many cells are damaged and where those cells are located in the brain determine the effect of the brain attack. Some people may experience paralysis, usually on the right side of the body. A brain attack also can affect an entire side or just a limb. Other people experience behavioral changes, and still others may not be able to speak, write, or even urinate.

Three kinds of brain attacks occur. The first is commonly referred to as a mini-stroke, but the actual term is a transient ischemic attack (TIA). The attack comes on suddenly and may last a few minutes (sometimes up to 30 minutes). During the attack, the brain's blood supply is diminished. The good news is that, even though your parent will appear to be having a stroke, a TIA is temporary and reversible. Your mom or dad may become dizzy, slump over, be unable to speak, or exhibit slurred speech, but then quickly returns to normal. This doesn't mean he or she is in the clear; a TIA precedes about one third of all strokes, and about half occur within the year. So take this as a huge warning and get your parent to a physician.

The second type of brain attack is known as an ischemic stroke. In this case, it's not transient, meaning it's not temporary. An artery carrying blood to the brain is blocked; the lack of blood and oxygen damages the part of the brain that didn't receive this dynamic duo.

The third type of brain attack is a hemorrhagic stroke. In this instance, blood and oxygen reach their destination; however, the vessel transporting its precious cargo of blood bursts and leaks into the brain, destroying brain cells in its wake. This type of brain attack is considered more dangerous and is involved in about 17 percent of strokes.

Sometimes physicians group ischemic and hemorrhagic strokes together and refer to them as a "cerebrovascular accident." Strokes are an emergency, and if treated quickly, some of the damage can be contained and even reversed. If given within the first three hours from the onset of symptoms of an ischemic stroke, an FDA-approved clot-busting drug tPA (tissue plas-minogen activator) may reduce long-term disability. So be sure to note the time of the first symptom and ask physicians attending to your loved one if the drug is appropriate for him or her.

The National Stroke Association identifies three warning signs of a stroke that warrant a 911 call. They created the acronym FAST to help you remember what to look for and what to do:

- **F**ACE: Ask the person to smile. Does one side of the face droop?

- **A**RMS: Ask the person to raise both arms. Does one arm drift downward?

- **S**PEECH: Ask the person to repeat a simple phrase. Is speech slurred or strange?

- **T**IME: If you observe any of these signs, call 911 immediately and record the time you saw these symptoms.

If you'd like a wallet card on FAST, go to www.stroke.org to download and print a copy. Given the high risk of strokes among older people, take the time now to identify which local hospitals nearest your parent have received certification as a Primary Stroke Center. The Joint Commission, the accrediting body for medical institutions, grants this distinction to hospitals that have made "exceptional efforts to foster better outcomes for stroke care." You can find the latest listing by going to www.qualitycheck. org. You may search by name, state, or zip code, and then at "Type of Service," choose "Stroke (Primary Care Center)."

Tip

The National Institute of Neurological Disorders and Stroke has an excellent website that provides information on brain attacks, symptoms, the latest research, and lifestyle advice. Visit www.ninds.nih.gov for more. The National Stroke Association hosts a site that identifies support groups and offers great resources for family members, at www.stroke.org; you can also call 1-800-STROKES (1-800-787-6537).

In addition to the FAST symptoms, the National Stroke Association also identifies other symptoms of a stroke that can come on suddenly:

- Numbness or weakness of the face, arm, or leg (especially on one side of the body)

- Confusion

- Trouble speaking or understanding

- Trouble seeing in one or both eyes

- Trouble walking

- Dizziness

- Loss of balance or coordination
- Severe headache with no known cause

Even though FAST doesn't cover every symptom, the vast majority of people will experience at least one of the three symptoms. It's a great way to remember what to look for during the chaos of an emergency when a precious three-hour window for a clot-busting drug is ticking away.

Cancer

Chances are, if you're reading this book, you are middle-aged and you've seen your fair share of family and friends struggle with a cancer diagnosis. Perhaps you've even fought your own cancer battle. I won mine against malignant melanoma, but my youngest brother did not. At the young age of 44, he left behind two young children within 12 heart-wrenching weeks of discovering he had cancer. Cancer is the second-leading cause of death in the United States. Among older people, cancers of the lung, breast, prostate, and colon are the top four.

Cancer is basically cells gone haywire. Their DNA message has been hijacked by cancer cells that then send errant messages so they can cleverly reproduce themselves. Some create tumors that stay to themselves—we call this type of cancer *benign*. But other cancers run amok, taking over organs and destroying their ability to function—these are malignant, and they are deadly.

The American Cancer Society has been warning us of cancer symptoms for decades: a sore that won't heal, changes in a mole or a wart, blood in the urine or stool, persistent indigestion or stomach discomfort, a sore throat that won't go away, a nagging cough, hoarseness or coughing up blood, unexplainable pain that won't go away, or a thickening or lump on any part of the body (especially the breast). If your mom or dad has any of these symptoms, it's really time for a doctor's appointment.

You might have to probe your parents for symptoms and urge them to make an appointment. When I made my rounds at senior centers as Secretary of Aging, I can't tell you how many times older women would tell me, "What you don't know, won't hurt you." They'd forgo mammograms, colonoscopies, and plenty of other cancer screenings, despite the fact that Medicare covers them. Many also felt that, if they had cancer, not much could be done anyway, so they didn't act fast enough and instead allowed their cancer to progress to later stages. Worse yet, they felt they were too old to prevent cancer, so they kept smoking or engaged in other poor lifestyles that the American Cancer Society warns against.

This sort of "magical thinking" flourishes among the geriatric set. Stay alert and encourage your parents to take advantage of the free screenings Medicare offers. Simply go to www.medicare.gov and click on the Resources Locator navigation bar. Check out the "Medicare & You Handbook" and enter the keywords "preventive services" in the search bar. You can print a checklist of all the free screenings and keep track of whether your parents have taken them.

Tip

The American Cancer Society (www.cancer.org) is the go-to website for everything you want to know about cancer. You can also find local support groups and information on more than 70 different kinds of cancer, or call 1-800-ACS-2345. The National Cancer Institute is also an excellent site to learn about cancer and available clinical trials. Go to www.cancer.gov or call 1-800-4-CANCER (1-800-422-6237).

Alzheimer's and Other Dementias

The new rage today is "brain fitness," geared especially toward worried baby boomers who don't want to become victims of Alzheimer's disease. They've watched dementia devastate the lives of their parents and grandparents and are hoping that breakthroughs in research, lifestyle changes, medications, and activities to keep their brains sharp will stave off the disease.

The term *dementia* is derived from Latin and means "without mind." It is a broad term that covers loss of brain function due to certain diseases. It steadily strips away one's ability to remember, think, speak, judge, and behave in ways that are considered normal. Recent studies suggest that people can have more than one dementia, and in that case, a loved one could be diagnosed with "mixed dementia." Most types of dementia cannot be reversed, causing brain damage that will continue to progress. It explains why physicians tell their patients that the disease is degenerative.

One of the most difficult conversations to have with a parent is whether to see a physician as a result of lapses in memory and judgment. Even if your parent has raised the issue with you, it isn't easy. My dear friend Joan approached me recently on this very subject. It was evident that something was going on with her mom: she'd forget that she had just discussed why friends would be leaving her dinner party early, but when they got up to leave, she acted surprised and asked why they were going so soon. She started to leave the front door unlocked, which she never previously did, and she'd interject stories into a conversation that had no real connection. Her mom was aware that something was amiss, but she was embarrassed and didn't want to talk about it.

I talked with Joan on how to approach her mother, and the following shows how Joan eventually convinced her mom to see a specialist. Joan's mother later allowed her husband to become part of her subsequent appointments.

Joan waited for what she felt was the right moment to talk with her mom and calmly told her, "Mom, lately you just haven't seemed like yourself." She didn't rattle off a list of mishaps her mom had made, as it would have caused her mother to feel embarrassed and defensive. Instead, she let her mom interpret what she meant by "not like yourself" and just waited for her reaction.

Her mom did admit that she wasn't feeling "like herself," but she didn't elaborate much other than to say that she had been forgetting things more than usual. She chalked it up to traveling and having been on the go too much. Joan took that as an opening and went a little further.

"That sure could be a reason … and I wonder, too, if it could be your medications, or maybe you have a vitamin B_{12} deficiency, which has been in the news a lot. I heard that might even cause people to feel confused." Joan was giving her mom options to consider and, for the first time, used the word *confused*.

By identifying a number of causes, Joan was also laying the ground-work for her next suggestion: "You know the best way to find out,

Mom, would be to see a doctor. The answer could be pretty simple. And even if it isn't, you've always taught me that it's better to act early." Her mom quietly responded with, "I know," and then changed the topic of conversation. Joan let it be.

A week later, Joan's mom called to let her know that she had set up an appointment. It took a number of other mishaps and conversations with her husband to encourage her to allow both of them to accompany her to the next appointment to go over the test results. Joan's mom also gave them permission to share with the doctor their observations and worries.

If you, your dad, or your mom is worried that they, a spouse, or a loved one may have dementia, intervening early can make a significant difference in their care and future. At the Alzheimer's Association website (www.alz. org), you can print a checklist of symptoms that act as a journal to describe what you or a loved one has been experiencing. This list will be a helpful aid during a physician's visit. The website also has a list of questions to ask the doctor, called "Preparing for Your Doctor's Visit." You can also give the association a call at 1-877-IS-IT-ALZ (1-877-474-8259). The website is a terrific resource, alerting you to the latest research, treatments, clinical trials, and loads of information for helping caregivers cope. I especially like the virtual tour of the brain, for an enlightening visual understanding of Alzheimer's as a brain disease.

Many people think that Alzheimer's disease is the only type of dementia. It is the most common, but there are many forms of dementia, and two in particular have a significant impact upon older people—vascular dementia and lewy body dementia. Let's go over the basics on all three.

Alzheimer's Disease

This is the most common cause of dementia in people age 65 years and older. However, young-onset Alzheimer's can strike 10 to 20 years earlier. In this case, the cause is most likely attributed to a defective gene. Researchers report that neuron damage is affected by plaques (deposits) and tangles (twisted strands) of the protein fragment beta-amyloid found among brain cells. It usually advances slowly, over 7 to 10 years, causing a steady decline in cognitive function. To track early indicators of Alzheimer's in your parent, check out the figure on the next page, which shows the Alzheimer's Association's 10 signs of Alzheimer's.

MISC.

Social Security Disability for Young-Onset Alzheimer's

If your loved one is diagnosed with young-onset, also known as early onset, Alzheimer's then they may qualify for Social Security Disability Income (SSDI). Recently, the Social Security Administration added early onset to its "Compassionate Allowance" list that identifies medical conditions that meet SSA's disability standards. This means the application process will be faster and payments will be rendered more quickly.

Vascular Dementia

Also known as "multi-infarct" or "poststroke" dementia, this type of dementia is the second most common dementia and occurs because of injuries to the brain caused by blood vessel blockage, bleeding, or other problems of arteries that affect the heart and brain. Symptoms begin suddenly, often after a stroke, and may occur in people with high blood pressure or who have had previous strokes or heart attacks.

Lewy Body Dementia (LBD)

This type affects approximately 20 percent of people with dementia and is more common with advancing age. "Lewy bodies" are abnormal clumps of protein similarly found in the brains of people with Alzheimer's and Parkinson's disease. The symptoms are similar to Alzheimer's disease, but its unique features are: sleep disturbances (e.g., kicking, thrashing), spontaneous confusion, visual hallucinations, and muscle rigidity and tremors akin to Parkinson's disease.

People with LBD exhibit more behavioral and emotional symptoms than those with Alzheimer's, and their motor impairments cause higher levels of physical disabilities. For these reasons, family members are faced with caregiving that is very demanding physically and exhausting emotionally.

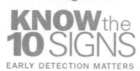

alzheimer's association·

KNOWthe
10 SIGNS
EARLY DETECTION MATTERS

Have you noticed any of these warning signs?
Please list any concerns you have and take this sheet with you to the doctor.
Note: This list is for information only and not a substitute for a consultation with a qualified professional.

____1. **Memory changes that disrupt daily life.** One of the most common signs of Alzheimer's, especially in the early stages, is forgetting recently learned information. Others include forgetting important dates or events; asking for the same information over and over; relying on memory aides (e.g., reminder notes or electronic devices) or family members for things they used to handle on their own. **What's typical?** Sometimes forgetting names or appointments, but remembering them later.

_____

_____

____2. **Challenges in planning or solving problems.** Some people may experience changes in their ability to develop and follow a plan or work with numbers. They may have trouble following a familiar recipe or keeping track of monthly bills. They may have difficulty concentrating and take much longer to do things than they did before. **What's typical?** Making occasional errors when balancing a checkbook.

_____

_____

____3. **Difficulty completing familiar tasks at home, at work or at leisure.** People with Alzheimer's often find it hard to complete daily tasks. Sometimes, people may have trouble driving to a familiar location, managing a budget at work or remembering the rules of a favorite game. **What's typical?** Occasionally needing help to use the settings on a microwave or to record a television show.

_____

_____

____4. **Confusion with time or place.** People with Alzheimer's can lose track of dates, seasons and the passage of time. They may have trouble understanding something if it is not happening immediately. Sometimes they may forget where they are or how they got there. **What's typical?** Getting confused about the day of the week but figuring it out later.

_____

_____

____5. **Trouble understanding visual images and spatial relationships.** For some people, having vision problems is a sign of Alzheimer's. They may have difficulty reading, judging distance and determining color or contrast. In terms of perception, they may pass a mirror and think someone else is in the room. They may not recognize their own reflection. **What's typical?** Vision changes related to cataracts.

_____

_____

____6. New problems with words in speaking or writing. People with Alzheimer's may have trouble following or joining a conversation. They may stop in the middle of a conversation and have no idea how to continue or they may repeat themselves. They may struggle with vocabulary, have problems finding the right word or call things by the wrong name (e.g., calling a "watch" a "hand-clock"). **What's typical?** Sometimes having trouble finding the right word.

_____

_____

____7. Misplacing things and losing the ability to retrace steps. A person with Alzheimer's disease may put things in unusual places. They may lose things and be unable to go back over their steps to find them again. Sometimes, they may accuse others of stealing. This may occur more frequently over time. **What's typical?** Misplacing things from time to time, such as a pair of glasses or the remote control.

_____

_____

____8. Decreased or poor judgment. People with Alzheimer's may experience changes in judgment or decision-making. For example, they may use poor judgment when dealing with money, giving large amounts to telemarketers. They may pay less attention to grooming or keeping themselves clean. **What's typical?** Making a bad decision once in a while.

_____

_____

____9. Withdrawal from work or social activities. A person with Alzheimer's may start to remove themselves from hobbies, social activities, work projects or sports. They may have trouble keeping up with a favorite sports team or remembering how to complete a favorite hobby. They may also avoid being social because of the changes they have experienced. **What's typical?** Sometimes feeling weary of work, family and social obligations.

_____

_____

____10. Changes in mood and personality. The mood and personalities of people with Alzheimer's can change. They can become confused, suspicious, depressed, fearful or anxious. They may be easily upset at home, at work, with friends or in places where they are out of their comfort zone. **What's typical?** Developing very specific ways of doing things and becoming irritable when a routine is disrupted.

_____

_____

If you have questions about any of these warning signs, the Alzheimer's Association recommends consulting a physician. Early diagnosis provides the best opportunities for treatment, support and future planning.

For more information, go to www.alz.org/10signs or call 877-IS IT ALZ (877.474.8259).

Getting a Heads-Up: Geriatric Assessments

According to the Centers for Disease Control and Prevention (CDC), the average person 65 years or older has two chronic conditions. The list of possibilities is pretty familiar: diabetes, hypertension, arthritis, heart disease, disabilities caused by a stroke, vision and hearing loss, lung disease, dementia, mental illness, and cancer. A chronic condition lasts a year or more, demands continuous medical attention, and often limits how an individual performs activities of daily living (ADLs).

Each condition comes with a specialist, a few medications, and a likely list of lifestyle changes. In no time at all, your parent may be taking six medications and seeing at least three to four different doctors, including a primary care doctor. You and your parents will be taking part in a medical juggling act that few of us are prepared to balance.

The physiology of an older body benefits from the expert eye and training of a geriatrician, a physician who has mastered the branch of medicine that diagnoses, treats, and prevents diseases and conditions among the elderly. A physician who is board certified in geriatrics has passed a national exam in the specialty and is attuned to the fragile state of an aging body. He or she knows how medications and their dosage levels affect older patients differently than younger ones, how various chronic conditions interact with each other, and how they should be managed. Geriatricians are familiar with the subtle signs of dementia and depression that a general practitioner may miss or misdiagnose.

If you're struggling to figure out what's wrong with Mom or Dad, if you or the physician suspect dementia, if your parent is struggling with two or more chronic conditions and is having difficulty doing so, and/or if your parent is taking multiple medications, a geriatric assessment is a smart route to take.

What's a geriatric assessment? A team of specialists from various disciplines perform exams and tests to assess an older person's health and functional abilities. They discuss your parent's findings as a group, with each sharing professional insights. Then they develop a comprehensive and integrated plan of care that includes input from the patient and family. The core team usually consists of a physician, nurse, social worker, psychologist, and pharmacist, all of whom have specialized in geriatrics.

Depending on problems your parent has presented, other professionals may join the team: a respiratory therapist may test lung capacity, an occupational therapist may evaluate your parent's ability to manage the tasks of daily living independently and safely, and a physical therapist may address your parent's physical limitations. If dementia is a concern, a neurologist and/or geriatric psychiatrist may examine Mom or Dad. Dietitians, optometrists, and hearing and vision specialists are also likely candidates for your parent's super team.

The search for a geriatrician may be difficult, as only 9,000 specialists are practicing throughout the entire country. Other than board certification in geriatrics, the American Board of Family Medicine with the American Board of Internal Medicine offer doctors a Certificate of Added Qualifications in Geriatric Medicine (CAQGM). Physicians who receive this certificate must have completed an accredited fellowship training program in geriatrics and passed a one-day computer-based Geriatric Medicine Examination. So if you're looking for a physician who trained in geriatrics, look for someone who is board certified or has received a CAQGM. Just because a doctor sees a lot of elderly patients in a practice doesn't mean he or she can use the title of geriatrician.

Tip	Call your local hospital to see if it offers geriatric assessments. Most university-based hospitals conduct them. You can also ask if the hospital has a list of physicians who are geriatricians. Another resource is the American Geriatrics Society website, at www.healthinaging.org. Go to "Request a Referral" to find a local geriatric physician, or call 212-308-1414 to have a list sent to you.

Healthgrades.com is a commercial website that identifies doctors who self-report that they specialize in geriatric medicine. Go to "Find a Doctor" on the home page and enter "geriatrics" in the search bar. When you click on the doctor's name, you'll see whether that doctor is board certified in geriatrics. When you call for an appointment, be sure to verify that the physician is board certified in this specialty.

Researching Medical Conditions

The internet has become a phenomenal resource for researching medical conditions. But it's also overwhelming. Just enter the name of any disease, condition, or symptom in your web browser's search bar, and you get hundreds of thousands of leads. Which do you choose? Who do you trust? How can you track down fast yet credible answers without spending precious hours in front of a computer screen?

As a general rule, websites with .gov, .edu, or .org—which signify *gov*ernment, *edu*cational institution, or *org*anization (usually a nonprofit) respectively—are sites that aren't selling anything. As a result, they don't have a commercial motive behind the information they report.

The following are the top three websites I recommend for researching medical conditions:

- **www.medlineplus.gov:** This megasite assembled by the highly regarded National Library of Medicine and the National Institutes of Health and other government agencies provides in-depth material on hundreds of medical conditions. You can check symptoms; look up medical terms; take interactive patient tutorials; view an illustrated medical encyclopedia; look up detailed information on medications, vitamins, and over-the-counter drugs; and find links to other trusted sites to learn more.

- **www.mayoclinic.org:** The Mayo Clinic has been a respected consumer resource for decades, and its website delivers a wealth of information, similar to Medlineplus. The site features a Symptom Checker that helps you identify potential health conditions, given the symptoms you enter. I especially like the "Tests and Procedures" section that clearly explains how to prepare and what to expect for a wide range of procedures. It's nicely illustrated with photos and diagrams; in some cases, you can even view videos.

- **www.NIHSeniorHealth.gov:** The National Institutes of Health has narrowed the information available on their other sites to focus on what's important for seniors. It has a handy function of enlarging text or choosing to listen rather than read. You'll especially like the video library that makes it easy to understand, for example, what actually happens during a stroke or heart attack. You'll also learn how to prevent, manage, and treat conditions with healthy lifestyle tips.

If you want to research a specific disease beyond the sites I've recommended here, look for national societies and associations (such as the American Cancer Society and the American Alzheimer's Association), most of which are nonprofit organizations dedicated to providing first-rate consumer information, research, and advocacy for patients.

Essential Takeaways

- You can turn phone calls and visits into subtle "checkups" by observing your parents' actions and behaviors, and by listening for signs and symptoms that could spell trouble.

- Aging is a dynamic process, and a physician who specializes in geriatrics is especially attuned to medications, chronic conditions, diseases, and treatments that are unique to older patients.

- A geriatric assessment conducted by a team of professionals among multiple disciplines that come together to assess your parent can be extremely helpful in determining what's really wrong and how to address it.

- One of the best ways to be an advocate for your parent's health is to become educated on medical conditions for which they have been diagnosed.

chapter 2

Defining Problems: Considering All Viewpoints

Understanding your parents' views on aging

Common motivators that influence emotional responses

Defining workable solutions for caregiving issues

Most of us are used to solving problems. We do it all day long—and some people even make a living at it. Problems large and small come at us; sometimes we can successfully handle them, and sometimes not. Some of us tend to ignore them until they've grown so large that there's nowhere else to turn but straight into them.

We use our problem-solving skills, however adept they may or may not be, in a wide range of caregiving situations. Rarely are they straightforward or simple. They involve a range of family members who may not see eye to eye on what needs fixing or whether fixing is even required. Parents who are desperately holding on to their independence may not be forthcoming on what's really going on, so well-meaning adult children work with inaccurate assumptions and information. To make matters even more interesting, an older person's health is very dynamic. As soon as one problem is solved and you've settled into a stable routine, it doesn't take much to change it up again.

This chapter and the next focus on how to effectively define and solve problems in the throes of caregiving. They also provide you with added insights on how behaviors are not always what they seem to be—for both you and your parent. You'll learn how to dig a little deeper and respond a little more kindly.

Appreciating Your Parents' Perspective

Chances are, your parents lived a pretty independent life and want to keep it that way. They grew up during the Great Depression and a war like no other, which forced them to become one of the most resourceful and productive generations in recent history. As a member of the "Greatest Generation," they uphold values of respect, authority, self-reliance, loyalty, and privacy. They believe in hard work and admire people who are disciplined and who don't complain or brag. They long for the days when you could "take a man at his word."

Tip

For a full understanding of how your parents think generationally, and how baby boomers think in kind, be sure to read Chapter 13. You'll get insights on why parents and their adult children are frequently at odds when it comes to caregiving decisions.

Given this backdrop of generational values, your parents' view toward aging will, in some ways, be different than yours. First off, they are experiencing it in ways no other generation has before. Medical technology, surgical advances, control of infectious disease, and healthier lifestyles have them testing the limits of the human life span. Reaching 100 years old is a milestone, for sure, but it's becoming more common by the day.

Even so, my parents and their friends don't seem to relish the idea of becoming centenarians. In their mid-80s, they are grappling with chronic conditions that aren't going anywhere, "too many doctors and pills," "too many aches and pains," and the constant low-level fear of losing their mind to dementia or losing their independence due to a fragile body.

Your mom or dad may feel plenty of other fears, too, and never articulate them to you because they worry you'll intervene or see them as vulnerable. But the fears are there and affect their everyday life. It's not uncommon for older people to fear falling, especially if they live alone. Some restrict their physical activity because of this fear. The problem is that this strategy causes them to become isolated, lonely, and out of shape, all of which make them more frail and more likely to do the one thing they fear—fall.

Fear of Falling Not Unfounded

The Centers for Disease Control and Prevention reports that, among older adults 65 years and older, falls are the leading cause of death due to injury. They are also the most common cause of injuries and hospital admissions for trauma. In 2009, 2.2 million older adults injured in a fall were treated in emergency departments, and more than 581,000 of these patients were hospitalized.

If Mom feels frail and vulnerable, she may find herself more fearful than in the past: for example, she may see teenagers walking toward her in the mall as a threat, with the intent to steal her purse. Dad may stop answering the door because he's afraid someone will rob him.

Besides worrying about falls and threats from the outside world, your parents likely worry about their bodies as they watch friends being diagnosed with cancer, dementia, or diabetes, or suffering heart attacks and strokes. They live in fear that this could happen to them or their spouse.

A constant dose of television doesn't help matters, either. Watching reality shows in which so many families appear to be dysfunctional or listening to a constant stream of unsettling and violent news can lead many elder viewers to think that the world has become a dangerous and unfamiliar place. As a result, some retreat and withdraw.

If they live alone and don't have a chance to interact with a healthy, functional outside world, their fears become all the more real, especially when they feel so vulnerable physically.

I don't mean to portray a doomsday view of aging. But if you've chosen to read this book, my guess is that your parent is grappling with health and lifestyle issues that have him or her concerned and have caught your attention. How both of you respond to changes in your parent's abilities—to see, hear, get around, organize life, drive, live independently, and manage health care—will define your relationships. And I'm talking not only about your relationship with your parent, but also about your relationships with your siblings, spouse, and children.

Deciphering What's Really Going On

No one likes to feel powerless. It throws us off balance and makes us uncomfortable. We'd rather opt for what's familiar and gain back the status quo. Fears that older people harbor and their diminishing abilities to function fuel feelings of powerlessness. Given their generation's strongly held values of independence and privacy, they may not be inclined to tell you how they're faring because they fear you'll intervene and they'll become even more powerless.

That's exactly why Doris, a dear friend of mine who lived alone and fell, didn't tell her daughter, who wanted her to live with her and her husband. If her daughter knew she had been unconscious for a half-hour and needed stitches from a nasty fall in her bathroom, Doris was certain that her daughter would use that as the "last straw" and make her mother move. My friend did realize, however, that it was no longer safe for her to live alone, for a number of reasons, and asked if I'd go "shopping" with her to find a senior living community.

Doris wanted to maintain control of her life and pre-empted her well-meaning daughter from making the choice for her. Once she found a place, she invited her daughter to look at it with her. She used that opportunity to tell her that this was where she planned to live because it really mattered to her to remain in the community where she had grown up some 85 years earlier. Even though her daughter would have preferred that she move in with her, she felt relieved that her mother had chosen an option that ensured her safety and gave her a vibrant life full of activities.

The driving force for Doris was maintaining control and staying independent. She also knew, without ever admitting it to her daughter, that her health and ability to live alone warranted a change. Doris's case turned out well, but in many instances, keeping secrets or not sharing what we really feel can place relationships and even lives in jeopardy.

Learning to dig a little deeper and understand what's really going on when you and your parent disagree over a caregiving issue is a skill worth learning. Let's give it a try by reviewing another true story; see if you can guess what each family member really feels.

Jake had been complaining of dizzy spells and was due to see his cardiologist later in the month. At the age of 90, he was generally in good health and had been his wife's primary caregiver for the past five years. Shirley was legally blind and could no longer manage her multiple medications. She also had severe neuropathy, causing her to lose her balance and fall without warning. Given her severe osteoarthritis, she had broken four different bones in the past five months. She continued to use a walker, although her daughters and Jake encouraged her to use a wheelchair.

Shirley recently fell and broke her shoulder. Jake had unintentionally been mixing up her medications and giving her sleeping pills in the morning, which contributed to the fall. Her orthopedic doctor prescribed using a home health aide to assist her when transferring from her wheelchair to the toilet, couch, and bed. The doctor also advised her to have someone assist her in taking a shower and recommended that a trained person do this instead of Jake while Shirley recovered.

Their daughter Kim, a nurse, flew out for a week to help. Before she left her parents, she made arrangements for a home health agency to send aides every day to assist her mother. She also arranged for a nurse to set up her medications once a month so that all Jake had to do was hand Shirley the set of pills in each compartment throughout the day. Shirley's long-term care insurance would cover the costs, so there was no expense. Jake and Shirley agreed with the arrangement and thanked Kim for coming out to help. In fact, Shirley was relieved that Jake wouldn't be responsible for sorting out her medications, as she felt it was getting too confusing for him.

By the time Kim got to the airport to fly back home, the agency had called her and said Jake had cancelled the service—and Shirley had agreed.

Let's pretend you're the daughter. If you'd gotten that call, how would you feel? Write out your first three reactions:

_____   _____   _____

I've used this case study for caregiver workshops, and the first reaction is an audible group groan. The participants rapidly blurt out these frequent responses:

Emotion	Digging a Little Deeper
Anger	How could my dad place Mom at risk for another fall? He's so selfish!
Shock	I can't believe they did this.
Resentment	I'll have to come back because she's going to hurt herself again.
Helpless	They are competent adults; what can I do if they don't listen?
Betrayed	They agreed to this. I can't believe they lied to me.
Scared	I'm worried about both of them. He seems more confused, and she's more fragile. I'm afraid for the future—theirs and mine.
Unappreciated	Don't they get what I did to come and help? I've lost vacation days and left my office mates in a bind. It took a lot to get everything organized for them.

Once everyone in the workshop has vented—they actually do get pretty upset with the parents—we spend time trying to figure out what motivated Shirley and Jake to cancel the service. What were their underlying feelings?

Here's what most workshop participants generally come up with.

Jake's underlying feelings are:

- He's feeling powerless and probably feels that his daughter thinks he's a failure.

- He's been in charge of Shirley's care and doing a good job—now he's suddenly not good enough?

- He takes pride in being her caregiver, and that's being taken away from him.

- He doesn't want strangers taking over or being in their home.

- He feels insulted and unappreciated, just like the daughter.
- He might be afraid that his health is failing and doesn't want to admit it by allowing help to come in.

Shirley's underlying feelings are:

- She doesn't want to hurt his feelings, so she lets him help her.
- She feels caught in the middle between her husband and her daughter, but since her husband's caring for her 24/7, she needs to go along with him.
- She's afraid that if she admits Jake isn't able to take care of her any longer, they'll need to move to assisted living.
- She doesn't want to admit to her failing health, so she'll keep things as they are—it makes her feel more independent.
- She's afraid of making Jake angry.

When you take the time to step back and give your parents the benefit of the doubt, to acknowledge that they aren't intentionally out to insult, ignore, or hurt you when they don't follow your advice, you'll be more open to understanding the emotions that underlie their behaviors. Calmly addressing "what's going on" and exploring potential solutions puts all of you in a better position.

But before we discuss strategies that can help you and your parents define caregiving problems, let's take a step back and consider some of the more common motivating factors that influence adult children. (In the next chapter, we discuss how to tackle these problems and solve them.)

Identifying Your Motivations and Emotional Triggers

According to experts and marketers who've studied this generation, baby boomers value flexibility, freedom of choice, self-improvement, expression of feelings, and success. They question authority. They've learned to multitask—perhaps not as adeptly as their smart phone kids, but they've learned to juggle careers and family in ways their parents never did. They view experts like physicians as knowledgeable consultants rather than godlike authority figures, in contrast to their parents' view.

Beyond these generational differences, you are your parents' child. That brings the most powerful layer of influence on how you view your parents and tackle caregiving issues.

If you have siblings, those relationships further affect your kaleidoscopic lens used to focus on the caregiving situation before you. For more on family dynamics, be sure to read Part 4 of this book.

When you find yourself bubbling up with a surge of emotions in response to a caregiving issue with your parent, steal away a few moments to dig a little deeper and sort through where these feelings are coming from. Here are some of the more common motivators that influence emotional responses from caregivers:

- **I must save them from themselves.** You feel responsible if anything goes wrong and believe your parents really don't know any better. Even if they do, they still must be rescued. You'll do whatever it takes, even if it means unrealistic sacrifices. You'll likely suffer from caregiver burnout and risk your other relationships because your self-sacrificing ways inadvertently ignore them.

- **Someone has to take charge.** You're used to making decisions and are likely the oldest child. People may defer to you at work and within your own family. You don't have time for a "wait and see" approach. You see a problem and just fix it. If your parents don't listen or your siblings are too slow to respond, you feel unappreciated and become angry. You might decide to just throw your hands up and walk away.

- **I'm a good son/daughter.** You find meaning in helping your parents and enjoy doing so. Caring for them gives you a chance to give back. You may believe it is your duty to be a good child and care for your parents. This may come internally from your own sense of well-being or externally from others' expectations. Some siblings who do not get along use the "good child" motivator to compete with each other just like they did as children. Unfortunately, their parents' needs get caught in the crossfire while the adult children fight over what's "best" for Mom and Dad.

- **No one listens to me.** You may feel that your parents don't see you as a grown adult, that they have you frozen in time as a teenager and don't view your advice as valuable. Or you may feel that they're trying to protect you from "grown-up" decisions. Your siblings may feel the same way. Perhaps you're the youngest or the middle child. When you do give advice and it's not accepted, you immediately think it's for these reasons.

If any of these scenarios sound familiar to you, whether for yourself or for another family member, they'll act as emotional triggers whenever turmoil or disagreement arises.

Your Body Has Something to Say, Too

Besides psychologically responding to caregiving issues, be aware that if you are juggling family and career demands, are fatigued from stretching yourself too thin, and need to tend to health problems of your own, your emotions will wear thin as well. Research confirms that caregivers often have weakened immune systems.

Let's imagine that Kim, the daughter in our story about Jake and Shirley, relates to the "No one listens to me" motivator. She's the youngest child, and even though she's a nurse, she thinks that no one in her family takes her seriously. Now imagine what she must feel when she gets the call that her parents have cancelled the service. All those emotions that everyone in the workshop said they'd feel would be doubled in intensity for Kim. She would easily call up her past history with her parents, and if her sibling sided with Jake and Shirley, she would be all the more angry, resentful, hurt, and frustrated.

Even if there's just one ounce of truth to any of these motivators for you, make sure you stay aware of them. When you know what's triggering a strong emotional reaction, you can better manage it. Otherwise, you may find yourself in an out-of-body experience watching yourself spin out of control. When you return to earth, it won't be pretty.

Defining the Problem

It might seem like a simple enough question, but when it comes to caregiving situations, there's rarely a simple answer. Seldom is only one issue at stake or one person involved. If anything, there are quite a few moving parts.

For example, your mom may have had a hip fracture; she's in the hospital and is being told that she'll be discharged in a few days. She could either recuperate at home with therapists coming to the house or go to a rehab center, which would be better for her. But she is the primary caregiver for your father, who has congestive heart failure; if she goes to rehab, no one will be there to look after him.

You would need to take off work and piece together your husband's schedule with outside help to care for your two teenaged sons. Another option is to hire help to tend to your father, but that would be costly. Your mom claims to want to go home, but you can tell that she's worried about being able to care for your father while she recovers. Your dad feels guilty wanting her to come home, so he tells her to go to the rehab facility and convinces himself that he can manage with someone coming in a few hours a day.

What do you do? Whose best interests need to be served? It might appear as a single problem—should Mom go home or to the facility?—but six lives are impacted at differing levels depending on whatever is decided.

As you'll learn in the next chapter, problems are better solved if they are broken down into manageable parts. And as you've discovered in this chapter, emotions influence how you'll see those parts. In some cases, you may turn a blind eye to the problem altogether.

No matter what caregiving predicament you're facing, taking the time to identify, clarify, and define a problem is key to developing workable solutions. If you don't start off knowing what you need to fix, you'll find yourself thrashing about reacting to all those moving parts and emotional triggers we've been talking about.

The following are the key steps to defining a caregiving problem:

- Does everyone impacted by the problem agree that there is one? If your parent doesn't believe there's a problem but you do, that's your *first* problem to address.

- Involve those who have a stake in how the problem is solved. Your parents, your siblings, and possibly your in-laws are likely participants.

- Gather information (results of medical tests, physician opinions, geriatric assessments, services and resource materials, insurance policies, observations by family members) to help you analyze the root causes of the problem.

- Determine how pressing the problem is to solve. If a safety issue is involved that places your loved one or others in danger, you need to intervene quickly and short-circuit the problem-solving process. On the other hand, you may conclude that giving your parent time to sort things out or taking a "wait and see" approach is the more reasonable course.

- Take the time to talk, ask, and listen to your parent, to further understand how he or she sees the problem. Probe for any underlying feelings that may be influencing or obstructing how your parent views the situation.

- Identify emotional triggers and motivators that may be preventing you or your siblings from objectively seeing what's really wrong and what needs to be addressed.

- Gain consensus among the group that the source of the problem has been accurately identified. For example, if your mom is acting confused, before you start coming up with solutions to deal with her "dementia," determine its source. Her confusion could be a side effect of a new medication, rendering some of your "solutions" unnecessary and erroneous.

Once your family feels comfortable having defined the caregiving problem, write it down in plain and simple terms. This will keep you on track while you go through the problem-solving process described in the next chapter.

Essential Takeaways

- Caregiving problems often involve grappling with deep-seated feelings and concerns over maintaining independence.

- Well-meaning sons and daughters may rush in to solve problems without having all the necessary information or their parents' permission to render solutions that are workable or acceptable.

- You may not always be aware of what's motivating your emotional response when your parent doesn't take your advice.

- Taking the time to clearly identify and define a problem will save you and your family a lot of headaches and heartache, and gives you your best chance to come up with solutions that really work.

- It takes real effort to be empathetic to what your parent is going through. Listen, be patient, and understand your own emotions before reacting.

chapter 3

Developing a Caregiver Game Plan

Assessing caregiving needs and the tasks of daily living

Defining your goals

Creating criteria to achieve solutions

Gauging your caregiver needs and the resources to meet them

Creating solutions that meet your goals

Caregiving sometimes falls to us in the midst of a crisis. Other times, we come by it slowly—we make a few calls regarding Medicare, we organize medications, we offer to get the groceries, or we go to a few doctor appointments. We just do what we have to do and squeeze caregiving into our schedule while juggling a job, a family, and "a life."

As a result, our caregiving rarely involves a well-thought-out plan. Who has the time to sit down and do one, anyway? And besides, your parent's needs are continuously changing. It's a moving target. So why bother?

However, it *is* worth the bother. There's some truth to the old adage, "A stitch in time saves nine." And if there's any period in your life when you want to make a few stitches to save many others later, it's right now.

We spent time in Chapter 2 defining problems. Now let's figure out how to work toward solving them. Let's develop a game plan that meets both your needs and your parent's.

Identifying Caregiving Needs and Tasks

Rarely is there a shortage of topics when it comes to identifying caregiving needs among older relatives. Social workers use extensive assessment tools to identify the needs of older clients and the level of help they need to address each. You'll hear geriatric professionals reference two basic categories: activities of daily living (ADLs) and instrumental activities of daily living (IADLs). The degree to which a person can perform these activities is used to determine whether an individual qualifies for different levels of care, such as assisted living, skilled nursing, or home health care. Long-term care insurance companies also use them to determine whether a beneficiary qualifies for certain services. ADLs refer to personal care activities that are essential to caring for oneself and maintaining independence. IADLs involve activities that are associated with the tasks and ability to live on one's own.

Tip

Go to www.lindarhodescaregiving.com and click "Resources" to download, save, and print Caregiving Task Assessment and Caregiving Resource Assessment Worksheets to help you complete all the tables and tasks described in this chapter. It's an easy way to keep track of the tasks you perform, what your parent needs, and the resources required. You can also use them to apprise other family members of what's needed and what they can do to help.

You can also download a Medical Biography form, a Med Minder List of all of your parent's medications, a contact sheet of all health-care providers, and an emergency medical contact form.

The ADLs and IADLs are usually rated on a scale to determine how much assistance is required—for example, no assistance, some assistance, or a lot of assistance.

The ADL and IADL lists, along with a simple rating scale, can help you identify and assess the caregiving needs of your parent. Access the form online at my website (www.lindarhodescaregiving.com) and view a hard copy in Appendix B.

Here's a listing of general adult daily living tasks to get you started:

Caregiving Task Assessment Worksheet Part 1: Adult Daily Living Tasks			
Task/Activity	*Level of Help Needed*		
	None	*Some*	*A Lot*
Bathing			
Sponge bath			
Shower			
Full bath			
Dressing (putting on clothes)			
Grooming (hair, shave, teeth)			
Assistance with walking (a person must help)			
Uses walker			
Uses wheelchair			
Uses cane			
Getting in and out of bed/chair			
Assistance with going to the toilet			
Incontinence care (adult briefs, catheter)			
Meal preparation (make the meal)			
Arrange food on plate, cut food			
Place food in mouth			
Medication reminder (hand the person pills)			
Medication organizer (sort/place pills in dispenser)			
Socializing—how much are they interacting with others?			

Now let's take a look at instrumental adult daily living tasks:

Caregiving Task Assessment Worksheet Part 2: Instrumental Adult Daily Living Tasks			
Task/Activity	*Level of Help Needed*		
	None	*Some*	*A Lot*
Shopping (for example, groceries, clothes)			
Light housekeeping			
Doing laundry			
Handling the mail			
Scheduling doctor's appointments			
Transportation (for example, driving)			
Managing medications (for example, ordering refills)			
Managing money (for example, paying bills)			
Handling household chores (for example, garbage, repairs)			
Handling health insurance matters			
Number of hours can be left alone			

After you've gone over the Part 1 and Part 2 Worksheets, take out the tasks that involve some or a lot of assistance. If your answer to "Socializing" was "None" or "Some," then include that as well. Most ADLs do not include this item, but I believe it is integral to a person's physical and mental well-being. Plenty of studies verify the positive effects that human interaction has on older people. It can even stave off dementia; thus, it should be considered a daily adult activity. These are the tasks that require attention.

Now take your complete list of tasks requiring some or a lot of attention and enter the tasks on the Caregiving Resource Assessment Worksheet illustrated here. You can also fill it out online and print it from my website.

Caregiving Resource Assessment Worksheet			
Task/Activity	*Time (Hours × Per Week/Month)*	*Resource (Person[s])*	*Cost Per Week/Month*

In the second column, identify how much time each of these tasks requires on a daily, weekly, or monthly basis. For example, your dad might need his medications organized, and you bought a 30-day organizer from the pharmacy. It takes you two hours once a month to sort and place the pills in each compartment. You also call him every day to make sure he takes his pills, plus you keep track of when he needs a refill and you pick them up at the pharmacy. You figure out that these three tasks involve at least another two hours every week.

Under the third column, identify who completes each task: Is it you? A family member? A friend? Someone you're paying? A volunteer? Your parent? No one?

Here's an example for Sharon, who cares for her mother, Claire, who lives alone.

Caregiving Resource Assessment Worksheet

Task/Activity	Time (Day/Week/Month)	Resource	Cost
Bathing (shower)	2 hrs (3x/wk)	Mom	$0
Shopping for groceries	3 hrs (1x/wk)	Sharon	$0
Organizing medications	1 hr (2x/mo)	Neighbor	$0
Taking to doctor visits	3 hr (2x/mo)	Sharon	$30
Paying bills	1 hr (1x/mo)	No one	$0
Handling insurance matters	1 hr (1x/mo)	No one	$0

After you've completed these steps, you'll have a pretty good assessment of your loved one's personal caregiving needs, along with the time, resources, and costs required to perform each of them. Tasks and activities for which the resources are minimal, too demanding, or unreliable are problem areas to solve.

Let's go over the example. Sharon, the daughter, is performing the bulk of the tasks for Claire. It's taking her about six hours every week. She works full time and has two teenagers at home. Those six hours a week have become more demanding to her. The neighbor has not been so well herself and missed organizing Claire's medications last week. Even though Claire has been taking showers by herself, when Sharon completed the chart, she indicated that it requires "some assistance" because Claire has been complaining of dizzy spells. Claire is resorting to sponge baths and would like Sharon to visit on weekends so she can help her with her shower.

Sharon has also noticed during her visits that bills have been piling up on her mom's desk, as have several insurance claims attached with letters asking for more information. No one seems to be handling them.

Clearly, the resources to help Claire are becoming demanding for Sharon. Claire taking showers on her own isn't safe or sustainable. Depending on a neighbor for such an important function as organizing medications has turned out to be an unreliable resource, at best.

In terms of costs, the only out-of-pocket expense is currently the $30 Sharon pays for gas to the doctor appointments, but it should also account for the six hours she takes off work—she loses $25 per hour, or $150.

Sharon has six problems to address, all of which require a game plan. And it all starts with defining a goal.

What's the Goal?

The answer to this question is essentially what you, your parent, and your family members want to achieve. Another way of crafting a goal is to ask yourself what a positive result will look like. Your goal is a desirable outcome that will solve a caregiving problem.

Let's review a problem that Lucy and her daughter Marie need to solve and explore a few goal statements to address it.

Lucy, recently widowed, is 85 years old and lives alone. She has macular degeneration and can no longer read prescription bottles. Her husband had always handed her pills to her throughout the day. After her husband died, Marie set up a simple system in which she placed her two medications in separate areas on the kitchen counter. However, Lucy was recently prescribed two additional medications and must take them at different times throughout the day. She tried taking the four prescriptions on her own but mixed them up and landed in the emergency room because of a drug overdose. Marie is her closest relative but lives an hour away and works full time.

Let's focus on how Lucy's vision disability places her at risk of incorrectly taking her medications.

The first step is to ask the question, what would a favorable outcome look like? The answer essentially becomes your goal statement. Here are two suggested goals for Lucy:

- Lucy will be able to take her medications accurately every day.

- Lucy will take as few medications as possible and will be able take them accurately every day.

Developing the goal sets the course for identifying subsequent solutions. Your parent may have a host of problems to solve. If so, it's best to categorize the problems that relate to each other instead of coming up with a global goal meant to fix all of them. Problems are easier to solve if you break them down; you can then better focus on the issue and identify root causes that lead to more appropriate solutions.

The previous two goal statements are straightforward; each requires a solution to ensure that Lucy will be able to take her medications safely every day. The second goal statement adds the caveat that she will take as few prescriptions as possible, to lessen the risk of medication errors.

Now let's go back to Sharon and her mom, Claire, who shares the same goal of wanting to take her medications safely. If Sharon does not feel she can visit on weekends and give her mother a shower, she will have an additional goal of, "Mom will be able to take a shower safely once a week without me providing it." This will require Sharon to come up with a solution that will be acceptable to her mom and will address Sharon's time constraints.

The goal-setting and problem-solving process should involve those who have a stake in the outcome—the foremost person being your parent(s). It also must involve other family members besides the primary caregiver— even those that live far away or those who haven't been very involved in your parent's care. You might think it's easier to ignore a sibling whose opinion you don't value or whom you consider argumentative, but if these family members have a relationship with your parent(s), they will surely express what they think. If they feel threatened or angered by not being asked to share their view, you've planted the seeds of conflict that will grow into a vine to strangle your best efforts.

Set Your Criteria for Your Solutions

Before you go about solving your caregiving issues, it's helpful to decide what criteria the solution should meet. These benchmarks are standards that the care receiver and caregiver agree upon. Agreeing on criteria makes it easier to evaluate each solution to see whether it measures up to the accepted expectations and criteria.

Universal criteria that most people adopt regardless of the circumstance or solution being considered are detailed as follows:

Our solution will ...

- Be safe.

- Be respectful.

- Promote independence at appropriate levels.

- Be acceptable to the person receiving the care.

- Be acceptable to the primary caregiver.

- Be affordable.

- Not endanger the caregiver or care receiver's physical and mental well-being.

You will likely identify other criteria that will be more relevant to your parent's circumstances and the unique needs of family caregivers. The following list might help you generate your own benchmarks to meet.

Our solution will ...

- Allow the caregiver to balance his or her family and work life.

- Not jeopardize the caregiver's job and/or marriage.

- Maintain the care receiver's privacy.

- Not isolate the care receiver from family, friends, and favorite activities.

- Consider the preferences of the care receiver.

- Not place undue debt or expenses on the caregiver or care receiver.

You'll reduce the risk of conflict if you and your family members take the time to think through the basic principles that you want your solution(s) to address. Do this *before* you start generating a whole series of solutions.

You'll likely reach an agreement on the criteria—everyone wants the care that a parent receives to be safe, to be good for the parent's mental and physical health, and to promote independence that's realistic.

This positive experience starts you on solid footing and helps everyone stay focused on what's best for the loved one and the caregivers. If a debate arises over a particular solution, you can measure it against your benchmarks and start weeding out options that don't pass the criteria test.

Sizing Up Your Life and Resources

After you've identified your parent's caregiving needs and the criteria that must be met for any solution to be workable, you'll need to take stock of the resources that you, your parent, and your family members can contribute. You'll also want to explore public and private resources that can meet your parent's caregiving needs beyond and in addition to your and your family's capacity to help.

The factor that most often has the greatest impact on a family member's ability to provide care is lack of time due to job obligations and commitments to family. You'll need to assess these time constraints when deciding what you realistically can do. This realization might force you to track down alternative ways to meet your parent's needs.

If you are the primary caregiver and you work, your time is likely limited. You might have a job that allows you some flexibility. When emergencies, surgery, or a hip fracture occurs, you can take a leave of absence covered by the *Family Medical Leave Act* (*FMLA*).

Definition

The **Family Medical Leave Act (FMLA)** is a federal law that protects you from losing your job when you need time to care for a seriously ill family member (spouse, parent, child, or self). Employers with 50 or more employees must allow their workers at least 12 weeks of unpaid leave to care for a family member. You must have worked for the company at least 1,250 hours over the previous 12 months. Your company is obliged to give you full health benefits during your leave, and you are entitled to get your old job back or another position with equivalent duties and the same salary and benefits when you return. You can break up the 12 weeks' worth of time as needed. For more information on the FMLA, go to the U.S. Department of Labor website at www.dol.gov (enter "FMLA" in the search bar), or call 1-866-487-9243.

Regardless of your circumstance, if you know you need time either during work or away from work, talk to your Human Resources department or your supervisor to determine how either can assist you in performing your job while you help your mom or dad. Survey research from the national Family Caregiver Alliance shows that 64 percent of caregivers are employed, and nearly three out of four of them rearrange their work schedule to accommodate the needs of their parents. So don't feel like you're alone when you reach out to co-workers and Human Resources staff to find ways to perform well at work and meet your caregiving duties. In fact, many companies today are becoming more understanding as their baby boomer workforce faces an unprecedented caregiving wave.

Sizing up your life also includes assessing your family commitments—If you have a spouse, how supportive is he or she? Does this mean you are spending considerable amounts of time away from home? If you have children, what are their needs? Do you find yourself missing events that upset them—and you? Are you feeling torn between your children and your parents? Are you finding that you feel overly stressed juggling caregiving with multiple roles? Only you can evaluate and answer these questions; they are worth asking so you can reasonably calculate whether you can sustain your role as a resource.

Creating Solutions

Now that you've identified your parent's needs, goals, and criteria, and you've assessed how pragmatic and appropriate your resources are among family members, you should have a list in hand that indicates some gaps between what your parent needs and what family members can address. And therein lies your problem list to solve.

Let's go back to Sharon and her mother, Claire. As you might recall, Claire would like to take a full shower at least once a week and also needs help organizing her medications because she has macular degeneration. Until now, Sharon has been able to carve out six hours a week doing her mother's grocery shopping and taking her to doctor's appointments, but the added work of organizing her medications and giving her a shower is placing too much of a burden on Sharon. She works full time and has two teenagers at home. Given the economic recession, Sharon is worried about taking any time off work. She and Claire had a long talk and agreed on these criteria for any solutions they would entertain:

- Claire will remain living independently at home.

- The medication solution will be reliable, safe, and easy for Claire to follow.

- Sharon will be able to dedicate six hours a week in caregiving tasks.

- Claire will consider outside help if it is affordable and she likes the aide.

- Claire values Sharon taking her to doctor's appointments and would like her to continue to accompany her.

Given these criteria, Claire and Sharon can explore a number of solutions:

- They could hire a nonmedical senior-care company to send an aide to help Claire bathe once or twice a week. Many of these agencies have a special two-hour rate of less than $40 to assist with bathing.

- Because Claire has been complaining of dizzy spells, Sharon will contact her primary-care physician to see whether an appointment is needed to review her medications, evaluate her blood pressure, and perform a physical to see what's going on.

- Now that Claire lives alone, she and Sharon will feel more secure if Claire wears a personal emergency response system (PERS) pendant or necklace. Sharon has asked her sister, who lives out of town, to research different models and plans.

- Instead of spending three hours doing grocery shopping every week, Sharon could order Claire's groceries online. They could be delivered, or Sharon could pick them up when she comes to visit her mother, to save on the delivery charge. That way, Sharon could spend more time visiting Claire than going up and down grocery aisles. She could also look into volunteer programs at local churches, synagogues, or the local high schools to see whether someone would be willing to pick up and deliver the groceries. Sharon could also ask her sister to make the orders online.

- Sharon found an automatic pill dispenser that she can organize only once a month. It signals an alert whenever Claire needs to take her medication and then dispenses exactly what she needs to take. The device even has a feature that will text Sharon if her mother didn't take the medication. She and her sister can pitch in to help pay for the cost, which makes it more affordable to Claire.

- Sharon has been concerned that her mother isn't getting out much since her husband died. She can talk to her mother about using a publicly funded transportation service for seniors to take her to church and the club she used to belong to.

- Sharon's sister can set up paying most of her mother's bills online and can handle all insurance claims and correspondence. Sharon can mail them to her whenever she sees them on their mother's desk.

As you can see from the list of solutions, there's a mix of resources: some require payment, others tap volunteers, another uses a publicly funded benefit, and two involve technology and assistive devices. Sharon also reaches out to another family member who lives a long distance but is within reach of the internet. She had never considered asking her sister to help, given that she lives in another state.

Tip

You can find a huge database of assistive devices, products, technology, and equipment online at ABLEDATA, a federal information clearinghouse sponsored by the National Institute on Disability and Rehabilitation Research for older people and those with disabilities. It includes a description of devices, consumer reviews, and contact data to purchase products. Go to www.abledata.com to see the vast collection of products, or call 1-800-227-0216.

Plan B

Before you consider your work finished, be sure to address one more solution: Plan B. What is your back-up plan if the primary caregiver is out of commission? If one of your parents, for example, is the primary caregiver and lives alone, a fractured hip, a heart attack, or even a bad case of the flu will place both of them in jeopardy very quickly. If you're the primary caregiver, your life can change at a moment's notice, too: kids and spouses get sick, and so can you. A health crisis with your in-laws could arise, and your spouse might have to be off taking care of them. Your job demands could increase, and you don't want to place your work in jeopardy. Think through the resources and arrangements you'll need to keep things humming along if the primary caregiver can't continue.

Today, thousands of resources are available to aid families in their caregiving. Of course, the trick is finding them without becoming overwhelmed. For a treasure trove of resources, check out Appendix A.

Essential Takeaways

- Solving problems involves identifying a series of action steps that can save you time and a lot of headaches later. Identifying activities of daily living and instrumental activities of daily living that your parent has difficulties performing helps you develop a game plan to address them.

- To determine a goal, ask yourself, "What will a positive result look like?" Your goal is a desirable outcome to solve a caregiving problem that's acceptable to you, your parents, and your family.

- Every solution should satisfy a set of criteria that your family agrees on. Test your solutions against these benchmarks to make sure they meet your needs and expectations.

- Be realistic in sizing up your ability and time to address your parent's caregiving needs. A wide array of resources is available with thoughtful and targeted research. It's worth the time to find them.

chapter 4

Getting Your Caregiving Plan Organized

Imagining "what if" scenarios

Creating a portfolio

Caring from a distance

Meeting with your family and delegating responsibilities

Communicating and sharing information

Regrettably, most of us wait until a crisis before we start thinking about caregiving issues facing our parents. But making high-stakes decisions while your emotions are in overdrive and time is clearly not on your side almost always guarantees poor and uninformed choices.

I encourage all families to take a number of proactive steps to make sure your loved one receives the best possible care when a crisis hits. It's also a way for your parents to prevent conflicts among you and your siblings, because no one will have to guess at what Mom or Dad wants when they're in no position to act for themselves.

But beyond emergencies, being organized for everyday caregiving lends you some control and saves time in both the short and the long run. Having ready important papers, phone numbers of doctors and home-care aides, and notes from all those calls you've made regarding insurance will make life so much easier. And so will knowing what your parents want.

Doing the Advance Work

One of the best ways to conduct the advance work of caregiving is to play out "what if" scenarios when your parents are not yet facing them. Imagining hypothetical situations is not nearly as stressful as the "real deal," and people are much less defensive because they aren't being forced to make an all-or-nothing decision on the spot.

Start the conversation by letting your parents know that you want to do what's best for them in the event they need help. And one way of doing that is to think in advance about *what if* something went wrong and you needed assistance. Tell them you'd like to go over a number of possibilities and start planning now. Ask whether they would mind if you took notes.

Here are some examples of "what if" scenarios:

- If you had a stroke and were told at the hospital that you needed to find a place to recuperate and receive physical therapy before you went home, where would you like to go?

- If you had a heart attack, what hospital would you want to treat you?

- If you had a stroke or, perhaps for some other reason, your doctors felt it would be wise for you not to live alone, where would you like to live?

- If you broke your hip and could go home from the hospital only if you had home health care, is there an agency you like?

- If you could no longer drive, how would you like to get to places? What places, events, and friends are most important to you?

- If you had cancer, would you want to try alternative treatment and/ or receive chemotherapy and radiation?

- If you needed end-of-life care, would you want us to call hospice? Would you like to be at home, if at all possible?

In going over the answers, you might discover that neither you nor your parents are sure of the best place to recover from a stroke, where to receive physical therapy, or what agency provides the desired home health care. Many people don't realize that hospitals focus on acute care and a short stay for recuperation. Discharge social workers will be handing your loved one a list of nursing homes that offer rehabilitation for people recovering from strokes and broken bones who have every intention of going back home.

As part of your advance planning, you and your parents would do well to visit facilities ahead of time so none of you will be scrambling to find a suitable center when your mom or dad is told to leave that cozy hospital bed the next day. Chapter 7 shows you what to look for, what to ask, and how to find quality facilities, home health-care agencies, and more.

You and your parents should also interview home health-care and non-medical senior care agencies and choose the one you like. Go through the process of signing them up, which might require completing a nursing assessment and filling out insurance forms and other paperwork; then if a parent ever needs any of their services, the process can be initiated with a phone call. You'll find this especially helpful if you are a long-distance caregiver.

> **Tip**
>
> My mom thought I was being overly protective when, during one of my Phoenix visits, I asked her to meet with a few home health-care agencies and choose one she liked. That way, if she ever got sick, I could call and have a nurse look in on her. Three months later, she came down with the flu, and even though I live more than 2,000 miles away, a nurse visited her later that afternoon and called to assure me she was okay. The agency sent an aide every day to take care of her, get her groceries and prescriptions, make chicken soup, and give her the care she deserved. It would have taken days to get an agency in to see her had she not signed on with the agency—and, in the meantime, the flu could have turned into something more serious.

Discussing the "what if" scenario of where your parents would like to live, in case a physician tells them that it's not wise to live alone any longer, helps explore whether they'd like to live with a family member, bring in live-in help, hire a full-time caregiver, or pursue assisted living. You could also explore whether they have thought of other reasons that would cause them to decide to move—to independent living, for example. This is the perfect time to elevate the discussion to another level and approach a sensitive topic that many people prefer to ignore.

When you're done with all your research, create a "rainy day" folder that contains your parent's wishes and the results of your "what if" scenario discussions. Share it with your parents and make sure they are in agreement. Get their approval to share it with other family members so that all of you will be on the same page when you all really need to be.

Setting Up a Portfolio

I can't believe the amount of paperwork I've amassed over the years for both of my parents. I have an expanding file for each of them that's bursting with medical data, insurance forms and correspondences, brochures from home health-care agencies, and loads of phone notes from all the calls I've made regarding their care. I keep certain key documents in a special file that I have immediate access to. Chapter 8 covers many of these documents, detailing how to gain access and complete them, so be sure to use this chapter as a resource.

Caregiver Portfolio Checklist

Here is what you need in your portfolio:

- ❏ A living will, also known as an advance directive, identifies your parent's end-of-life care wishes.

- ❏ A durable health-care power of attorney is broader than a living will. It empowers you to make health-care decisions on your parent's behalf any time he or she is incapacitated.

- ❏ Power of attorney provides for specific powers granted to an agent (for example, a family member or friend), such as paying bills, selling property, or making other non-health-care-related decisions under certain conditions spelled out in the document.

- ❏ A contact list of physicians, home care and home health-care agencies, family members, significant persons, and agency services. You can access the Master Contact List form online at my website (www.lindarhodescaregiving.com) and view it in Appendix B.

❏ Emergency medical data, including a listing of allergies, health conditions, and family and doctor contact information, to be given to paramedics. You can access the My Medical Data form online at my website and view it in Appendix C.

❏ A medication list identifying all current medications, including over-the-counter medications, what each medication is prescribed for, and daily dosage level. You can access the Med Minder form online at my website and view it in Appendix C.

❏ A medical biography that details allergies, health conditions, and significant surgeries and procedures, including notes that describe any complications and family history of major health problems. You can access the Medical Biography form online at my website and view it in Appendix C.

❏ A numbers card that has your parent's important numbers that you'll most likely be asked: birth date, Social Security number, Medicare number, Medigap policy number or Medicare Advantage number, Part D Plan number, and any other insurance policy numbers. This card should not be in a folder that agency providers or other help visiting the home could gain easy access to.

You or someone else in the family should know where to find all the other important papers, including financial information, the will, and passwords for accounts and computers.

Long-Distance Caregivers—More Advance Work

If you live a long distance from your parent, beyond making plans for "what if" scenarios, you can take other actions to create an on-the-ground support system to alert you to problems or allow you to quickly kick into action. Having a plan buys you precious time if you have to rearrange work schedules, make arrangements for your kids, and travel to reach Mom or Dad in a crisis.

Next time when you visit, try some of these strategies:

- **Get to know the neighbors.** You'd be amazed by how much neighbors do for each other. On your next visit, go over to the neighbors' and share your contact information and ask for their phone number. If you're lucky, these are folks who knew you when you were growing up; even if you don't know them, ask them to check in with you if they become concerned about your parent, especially if he or she lives alone. Stay in touch with them, even if it's just a matter of sending them cards on the holidays.

- **Get to know the mail carrier.** Now, here's someone who probably knows more about your parent's routine than you do. For many older people, getting the mail is the highlight of the day, and they wait for a quick chat along with their mail. If Mom's not there, if she seems disoriented, or if her mail piles up, her mail carrier might pick up the warning signs and take action. If you'd like the mail carrier to pay a little extra attention, contact your parent's local post office and ask to sign your parent up for the Carrier Alert Program. If the mail carrier has any suspicions that something is wrong, he or she will then notify a supervisor, who, in turn, will contact a local partner agency (usually the Area Agency on Aging). The agency will check on your parent and contact you if there's a problem. Not all postal service offices have the program, so you'll need to ask.

- **Get to know the bankers.** It's probably a good thing that many parents are part of a generation that hasn't taken too fondly to automatic teller machines. An ATM sure won't give you a call that Mom just took out a large sum of money or that a stranger has been accompanying Dad to the bank. Introduce yourself to the bank manager and ask him or her to alert you of any concerns.

- **Draw up a phone schedule with your siblings.** A friend of mine happened upon an idea to keep up with his mom who lives several hours away. He noticed that when he talked to her on Sundays, she'd often just heard from his sister and brother, too. Instead of getting a triple dose of her kids in one day, he thought it would make more sense if each of his siblings agreed to call on separate days throughout the week. Now their mom gets a call just about every other day from one of them, which is more rewarding for her and provides a frequent checkup on how well she's doing.

- **Get to know your parent's best friends.** Your parent's friends can let you know if something's amiss and suggest that you should look in on your parents. My mother lives in Phoenix, and I've gotten to know her buddies pretty well. We've shared phone numbers, and one of them emails me. I try to stop by and say hello when I'm out there. Friends are your best eyes and ears, and they'll likely have your parent's best interest at heart.

- **Get to know the Area Agency on Aging.** See what the local Area Agency on Aging offers in your parent's community. This organization can help you track down a host of human services for your parents. To find the agency in your area, call the Eldercare Locator at 1-800-677-1116 or go to www.eldercare.gov. If you don't use the internet to track down local vendors and phone numbers, the next time you're visiting your parents, bring back an extra copy of the local phone book. You'll find the Yellow and Blue Pages of government and social agencies especially helpful. If you're online, you can always check out www.yellowpages.com.

- **Get to know your parent's religious community.** If your parent belongs to a church or synagogue, be sure to attend a service when you're visiting and introduce yourself to the religious leader. Many times, the group will have a social gathering following the service; attend it so you'll get to know your parent's circle of friends at church or synagogue. If your mom or dad is hospitalized or sick, be sure to call the priest, rabbi, or minister so she or he will pay a visit and let the congregation know, too.

If you're the primary caregiver because you live closest to your parent, there are still plenty of things your out-of-town family members can do to assist in your parent's care.

Family members can handle the insurance work by doing the following:

- Calling the plan's representatives when there's a dispute

- Filing claims

- Making sure premiums are paid

- Managing the annual sign-up period for Medicare

- Scheduling doctor's appointments

- Calling in prescription refills

- Making reminder calls to your parent to take his or her medication

- Paying bills and helping research any of your mom or dad's medical conditions

- Pitching in to cover the costs of providing assistance for nonmedical senior care that would provide you some respite

- Giving Mom or Dad gift certificates for home-delivered meals, cab rides, or a cleaning service (all of which would assist you, too)

Essentially, anything that involves simply using the phone or the internet is an ideal task for long-distance family members.

Delegating Tasks and Family Meetings

The most frequently reported frustration among caregivers is the lack of consistent help from other family members. In the National Family Caregiver's Association annual survey, three out of four family members repeatedly reported feeling this way.

Instead of counting on a "look at what a martyr I am" approach to throw your sisters or brothers into guilt-ridden action—or, more likely, defensiveness—start by asking them to help you go through the Caregiving Task Assessment and Caregiving Resource Assessment Worksheets you completed in Chapter 3 and to provide input on how all of you can share in the care of your parent.

One way of working through how each family member can assist with caregiving tasks and developing practical solutions is to hold a family meeting. Let's go over some pointers on how to convene one with win-win results.

Holding a Family Meeting

Caregiving should never be a solo act, especially if you have siblings and other extended family members. Many caregivers report, whether intentional or not, that most of the caregiving falls on them. But it doesn't always have to be that way. Sometimes you need to reach out to siblings, letting them know the caregiving needs of Mom or Dad and asking for help. Even siblings who live far away can help, as you've already learned.

One way of getting everyone to see and respond to Mom's or Dad's needs is to call a family meeting. For some families, this is a pretty normal process—everything's a group decision. But for others, it might seem too formal or even threatening. Not all family members get along, so including everyone in the same room could make matters worse. In that instance, you might serve as the broker and speak to each of them separately, to gain their input on how they can help and solicit their opinions on strategies that the entire group is considering.

> **Tip**
>
> Before you venture forth, remember that each of you has a different relationship with each of your parents, different life experiences, and, thus, different perspectives on how to handle his or her care. If one of your parents is the primary caregiver, the situation can become even more complicated because he or she is juggling the relationship with their spouse, you, and your siblings.

Now that we've gone through the process in Chapter 3 of learning how to define problems, identify caregiving needs and tasks, set criteria for successful outcomes, and develop goals to meet your parent's needs, you're prepared to bring your siblings together with your parent to map out a joint game plan. A family meeting can be an extremely helpful process to make that possible.

Who attends? The general rule of thumb is that everyone who has a stake in the care of the loved one should be present. This usually means siblings, the spouse, and the person receiving the care. If in-laws are close and usually participate in other family decisions, including them might be appropriate, too. You might also have a relative or family friend who is a nurse, a lawyer, or a professional in another relevant field that could be helpful. If all of you can't get together in one place, it's worth setting up a conference call. If your family is small enough, you can easily do an inexpensive three-way call or use Skype (www.skype.com), which is a free online phone/video service for those who sign up.

Who facilitates? One family member should be in charge of organizing the agenda and keeping the discussion on task.

But if your family has unresolved conflicts that will undoubtedly erupt in a meeting, look for a professional facilitator to hold the family meeting. A natural for this job is a geriatric care manager (see Chapter 6) or a social worker, psychologist, priest, rabbi, or minister. If everyone pitches in to pay for someone, the experience will be well worth it and affordable.

Meeting Preliminaries

If you're holding the meeting on your own, here are some suggestions for a productive family meeting:

- **Do your homework.** If you've gone through the process laid out in Chapter 3, you'll have the information you'll need to craft an agenda. It's helpful to share your Caregiving Task Assessment and Caregiving Resource Assessment Worksheets ahead of time and ask your siblings to add their thoughts to each. Ask if they have any other information that can enlighten the group's collaboration at the meeting, such as medical reports, research on health conditions and medications, and contact data regarding potential resources for help. Someone should also tackle bringing together your parent's financial and insurance information, to address discussions of cost issues for performing the caregiving tasks you identified on the worksheets. If housing options are to be considered, gather resource information on that as well.

  The goal is to have objective, relevant, and accurate information in front of the group so your family can make well-informed decisions. It also lessens the likelihood of emotional responses that might be irrational, given the situation being addressed. For example, a youngest daughter might not want to accept that Mom has Alzheimer's and can no longer be left on her own. She might try to refute anecdotal stories from an older brother, but a geriatric assessment from a reputable medical center is hard to argue with.

- **Create an agenda.** All family members should identify the two or three most important things they would like to discuss at the meeting and identify what they hope to see achieved as a result of the meeting. Chances are, you'll find overlap among family members, and this information will help all of you when it comes to setting goals and solving problems. It will also help set and clarify expectations.

Sample Agenda

An agenda could look like this:

1. Review what all participants want to accomplish, to address everyone's expectations. Identify a common overall goal for the meeting, such as, "We're here today because we want to work as a team to help Mom. By the end of the meeting, we'll walk away with a plan that works for her and is doable for all of us." Keep it simple. This is not the goal for solving specific problems; it's just a generalized, ideal goal for the meeting itself.

2. Review Parts 1 and 2 of the Caregiving Task Assessment Worksheet (see Chapter 3). Is there anything to add or subtract? Gain group consensus.

3. Identify all areas on the Caregiving Task Assessment Worksheet that indicate either some assistance or a lot of assistance needed. Enter all these on the Caregiving Resource Assessment Worksheet (see Chapter 3).

4. Gain consensus on the Caregiving Resource Assessment Worksheet.

5. Set your goal. What will a desirable outcome look like if you address the areas where resources are needed?

6. Set the criteria for your solutions to meet (see Chapter 3). Gain consensus—and be sure to write these down so the group can refer back to them throughout the discussion. If you find the group debating a solution, look back at the criteria—does it meet your benchmarks?

7. Now start your problem-solving session. Review the Caregiving Resource Assessment Worksheet. Wherever there are blanks (meaning that no one is currently addressing the problem or that the resource is limited, stretched, or unreliable), those are your problems to work on.

Rules of Engagement

Chances are, most of you have been part of a meeting that followed the basic Robert's Rules of Order. You don't need to be that formal, but ground rules do help when the topic can become rather emotional. Hopefully, these suggestions will guide your family toward a productive meeting about caring for your mom or dad:

- Follow the agenda that you all agreed upon.

- No cutting in—wait to speak until someone finishes talking.

- Don't hurl accusations, as in, "You always side with him."

- When you have something to say, it should reflect what you think, not what you think others think. So start the sentence with "I ...."

- Stay focused on your parent's needs. Rally around what's best for him or her, which means leaving old scores behind; it's not about you.

- If you're not clear on a point that your sibling has made, ask for clarification. Don't stay silent or assume that he meant something he didn't.

- If you want to make sure you've understood someone, try something like, "This is what I heard you say (then repeat what you think you heard). Is that right?"

- Create next-action steps as you complete each item on the agenda. Identify any other information you need to gather to make a more informed decision.

Wrap up the meeting with everyone clearly understanding what you have decided as a group. Identify who is responsible for what going forward. Create a list of those duties and share it before you disband.

When you and your siblings agree to a plan, make copies of it so that all of you have it. Be sure to update it as your parent's needs change. I also recommend setting up a convenient, weekly phone conversation to review your parent's care—that way, you'll form a partnership among you.

Social Networking and Online Information Sharing

Functioning as a team makes it much better for your parent and easier for all of you to work in unison. If all of you have internet access, take advantage of the convenience to exchange information on websites, send pertinent attachments, and email each other and any staff in charge of your parent's care. You could even set up your own secure Facebook page to share thoughts, ideas, and resources. Some caregiving and elder care websites enable families to share information with each other. CarePages, a free service at www.carepages.com, is especially helpful during a serious illness. A growing number of e-health personal health record platforms also is available online. We review these in Chapter 9.

This will be a challenging time for all of you, but if you openly communicate with one another, then anxiety, guilt, anger, and frustration are less likely to sabotage your relationships and your caregiving.

Essential Takeaways

- Unplanned decisions are uninformed decisions; in the heat of a crisis, they are rarely in anyone's best interest.

- Playing out "what if" scenarios provides a hypothetical, safe way to imagine what to do if an unexpected health-care crisis arises.

- Siblings and other family members who live far apart from parents can still assist with a wide range of caregiving tasks.

- Productive family meetings don't just happen. You need to plan them by assessing tasks, needs, and resources; forming an agenda; following ground rules; and applying the problem-solving format presented in Chapter 3.

chapter 5

Managing Your Stress

Understanding the toll stress has on you and your body

Assessing your stress: take the quiz

Uncovering what's really going on with your emotions

Getting a handle on your stress

Taking a break from caregiving

Finding support

Before we begin this chapter, let's start on a positive note: caregiving often is very rewarding. Most caregivers are generous souls who find meaning and purpose when they give of themselves. Many adult children welcome the opportunity, even though it might be under sad circumstances, to give back to their parents. But as you learn in this chapter, there is a toll.

According to a slew of studies, the typical caregiver is a 49-year-old married woman with a full-time job, kids at home, and the task of caring for a widowed mother who lives alone. She's arranging doctor's appointments, helping with her mom's tasks of daily living, and finding ways to make it possible for one or both parents to remain at home as they struggle with chronic and limiting health conditions.

Women in their 70s are caring for their older spouses, and for some, also caring for their parents, who are in their late 80s and 90s. Men, too, are joining the caregiver ranks and now make up one third of all caregivers, many of whom care for a frail, ailing wife. Older caregivers also struggle with their own health issues; in fact, one third report that their health is either fair or poor.

All are among the nearly 44 million Americans who care for an older loved one, according to the National Alliance for Caregiving. And virtually every one of them feels some level of stress. Let's talk about it.

Understanding the Toll of Stress

Even though I'll be citing studies that show the stressful side of caregiving, research also suggests that the act of helping people triggers hormones such as oxytocin that are known to promote cellular repair and cell growth. In research conducted by University of Michigan lead investigator and psychologist Stephanie Brown, adults 70 years and older who provided "14 or more hours of care per week to a spouse had lower rates of mortality than those who did not provide any care to a spouse." As it turns out, generosity and compassion are good medicine.

But what happens when the levels of care and the circumstances surrounding it become extremely difficult for long periods of time?

Stress isn't evident only from a few close friends confiding that you "don't look so good" or your spouse and kids grousing that you act "stressed out." Your body has plenty more to say on the matter; the trick is to know how to listen.

Our bodies are designed to react to stress. As soon as we perceive a threat, our nervous system releases a flood of adrenaline, cortisol, and other hormones to help us spring into action. We're more alert, our heart beats faster, our senses are sharper, our muscles are stronger, and we suddenly have more strength than we ever imagined. It's the formula for the "fight or flight" response that protects us from harm. This reaction can save your life. But it's also meant to be short lived.

When our bodies are overloaded with hormones reacting to stress, whether it comes in frequent bursts or in a steady stream, a deluge of physiological changes occurs. And instead of saving your life, stress can strip it away.

Multiple studies have shown that the risk of death is higher among care-givers, especially if they also suffer from a chronic condition. Studies led by Dr. Richard Schulz, professor of Psychiatry at the University of Pittsburgh, found that older spouses who reported caregiver stress had a 63 percent higher risk of death, compared to peers who had no caregiving role. And those who had a severe chronic condition died within the study's four-year follow-up.

According to Schulz and others, people who provide heavy caregiving duties suffer from depression, poor self-care, weight loss, and chronic ill-ness, and consider themselves in poor health. It's no wonder they decline more rapidly under the stress of caregiving—no matter how compassionate they might feel.

Alert	Researchers at the University of California at San Francisco zeroed in on the cellular level to see how stress affects the body. Dr. Elissa Epel found that chronic stress actually shortens the life of a cell. That leads to premature aging, which, in turn, can shorten a person's life up to an entire decade.

And there's more: scientists have found that stress causes a spike in a substance known as IL-6, a protein that weakens the immune system. Stressed-out caregivers thus are at high risk for infections, influenza, diabetes, cancer, and heart disease.

One study monitoring elderly caregivers found that their IL-6 levels were four times higher than those of their peers who reported less stressful lives. As we age, our IL-6 levels naturally rise, making the caregiver stress factor all the more alarming. Beyond IL-6 levels, the chronic activation of the body's fight-or-flight response system overexposes it to cortisol, the pri-mary stress hormone that produces sugar in the bloodstream. This alters the immune system, suppresses the digestive system, and affects the region of the brain that controls mood, motivation, and fear.

What's the bottom line? Plenty of research and just good old common sense forewarn that stress day in and day out can't be a good thing.

So why aren't more people alarmed? Why is caregiver stress so rampant? One reason so many caregivers don't detect feeling "stressed" or see it as harmful is that they just assume that the fatigue, headaches, back pain, and depression they feel are just part of the caregiver package. They become so familiar with feeling stressed that it starts to feel normal for them. Significant numbers of caregivers (nearly half, in some studies) also report having chronic illnesses themselves. The symptoms of illness and stress become so blended that they view them as just one in the same.

So let's get stress on your radar screen before it quietly steals away your health, your well-being and, in its extreme, your life. Familiarize yourself with the common symptoms that too much stress can cause.

Caregiver Strain: The Signs of Stress

Feelings

- Sad, unhappy, or depressed
- Short-tempered, easily angered
- Prickly, irritable
- Moody, temperamental
- Lonely, isolated

- Agitated, can't unwind
- Impatient
- Guilty
- Resentful

Thinking

- Unfocused, lack of concentration
- Faulty judgment
- Forgetfulness, poor short-term memory
- Incessant worry

- Racing, uncontrollable thoughts
- Inability to learn new information
- Negativity

Physical

- Fatigue
- Shortness of breath, chest pains

- Muscle and joint aches and pains
- Stomach pains, nausea

- Headaches, dizziness
- Tightness or knot in throat
- Impaired sleep
- Loss of sex drive

- Increased or decreased appetite
- Increased smoking, drug, and/or alcohol use

The good news is that you can feel these symptoms, and family and friends can call them to your attention. But you're also capable of denying them or becoming defensive. The bad news is that the bodily harm stress causes lurks beneath the surface, leaving you unaware of the damage it's doing to your organs, tissue, bones, and cells. Without addressing the stressors affecting your caregiving, you're at risk for significant health and medical problems. Among them are these:

- Hypertension
- Cancer
- Depression
- Heart disease
- Sleep disorders
- Digestive disorders

- Obesity
- Diabetes
- Autoimmune diseases
- Skin conditions (eczema, psoriasis, and shingles)

If you are diagnosed with any of these listed conditions, don't assume that it is unrelated to caregiving. It might not be the only factor, but it certainly does contribute. Facts compiled by the Family Caregiver Alliance report that nearly one out of every four caregivers who have been providing care for five years or more report that their health is fair or poor. Half to 70 percent have clinically significant symptoms of depression, and persons caring for someone with dementia will find their immune system compromised for up to three years postcaregiving. Cancer, high blood pressure, and heart disease have long been associated with stress as a mitigating factor.

You owe it to yourself to dig a little deeper to see just how much caregiver strain affects your life.

How Stressed Are You?

If I had to choose just three words to sum up how I feel while caring for my parents at a long distance or when I cared for my husband's grandmother who lived with us, it would be "torn in two." I always want to do more for them, but I also have a job, children, a husband, and others who need me. It's a feeling that plenty of caregivers share, and I've heard it from my readers in the form of a number of questions:

- "If I take vacation days to care for my dad while he recovers from knee surgery, will I have enough left to spend with my kids and husband?"

- "How do I make time for my marriage, between caring for two kids and caring for my parents?"

- "Do I go to my daughter's soccer game or take my mom to her doctor's appointment?"

- "I understand why my mom wants to live alone, but I spend 20 hours a week to make it possible. How long can she expect me to keep this up?"

- "Why do I feel guilty all the time? I'm stretched so thin, I feel like I'm letting everybody down—and that includes my health."

- "My friends tell me to take care of myself—do you mind telling me when?"

If you've asked yourself similar questions, then you're clearly among the millions of caregivers who are trying to balance their families, jobs, and lives while caring for loved ones, too. It can be done, but as the flight attendant directs you before take-off, "If we lose cabin pressure, place the oxygen mask on you *first,* then help your children." It's time to find out if you're low on oxygen.

A colleague of mine, Dr. Steve H. Zarit, a professor of human development at Pennsylvania State University, has written and researched extensively on caregiver stress and depression, especially among those who are caring for a loved one with dementia. He developed what is known as the Zarit Burden Interview, a questionnaire that has been used in hundreds of research studies and by physicians who want to learn how their patients are faring as caregivers. Dr. Zarit has allowed me to share his survey with you so that you can gain personal insights on the level of stress you might be experiencing as a caregiver. We use a shortened version of the interview tested and researched by Dr. Michel Bédard, Canada Research Chair in Aging and Health at Lakehead University.

The Short-Version Zarit Burden Interview

At the end of each statement, enter the number from the following answer key that best reflects how you feel:

Never	0
Rarely	1
Sometimes	2
Quite Frequently	3
Nearly Always	4

DO YOU FEEL …

1. Because of the time you spend with your relative that you don't have enough time for yourself? ____

2. Stressed between caring for your relative and trying to meet other responsibilities (work/family)? ____

3. Angry when you are around your relative? ____

4. Your relative currently affects your relationship with family members or friends in a negative way? ____

5. Strained when you are around your relative? ____

6. Your health has suffered because of your involvement with your relative? ____

7. You don't have as much privacy as you would like because of your relative? ____

8. Your social life has suffered because you are caring for your relative? ____

9. You have lost control of your life since your relative's illness?   ____

10. Uncertain about what to do about your relative?   ____

11. You should be doing more for your relative?   ____

12. You could do a better job in caring for your relative?   ____

Total Score: ____

Now add all the numbers. If your total is 0 to 8, your caregiver burden level is Low. If it is 9 to 16, it is Moderate. If your total is 17 or higher, you are likely experiencing a High level of stress, and it would be wise to address it as soon as possible. It might also be helpful to see your primary care physician and talk about your stress and any symptoms you may be experiencing. If your score is in the Moderate range, follow the suggestions and coping strategies discussed in this chapter and throughout the book. You really do owe it to yourself—and if you think you don't, read over the "Caregiver Covenant" section at the end of this chapter every day. I also recommend taking this inventory every month to monitor your stress level. All that being said, the Zarit Burden Inventory is not a diagnostic tool, nor does it take the place of your physician's opinion. It's a tool that can help you personally evaluate and reflect upon some of the strain you might feel as a caregiver.

Caregiver Emotions: Breaking It Down

Remember that list of emotions that caregivers commonly report feeling? Sometimes it's helpful to take a step back and dissect what's really going on so you can identify whether a certain pattern or trigger is sending you down an emotional path you wish you'd never taken.

Let's take a step back and review five of the usual stress suspects that just about every caregiver feels at one time or another.

Guilt

What's going on? Guilt is feeling badly about being responsible for some real or imagined wrongdoing. When it comes to caregiving, guilt often arises from all the "should haves": we should have taken Mom to the doctor sooner, spent more time with Dad, not been so impatient, or had things better organized. Probably the greatest contributor to guilt is making that classic promise to never place a loved one into a nursing home. If you break it because you totally underestimated the level of care your loved one would require, you feel guilty. And if you keep the promise and provide care beyond what you expected and have twinges of anger, frustration, or resentment for having made the decision, you still feel guilty for secretly wishing you'd never made the promise.

Guilt can also be externally imposed by a parent who reminds you of "all I've done for you," with the implied *quid pro quo* that now it's your turn. It's also spun from wanting to be a good daughter or son, in terms of both internal expectations and those from friends, family, and society. "Honor thy father and thy mother" runs deep.

How should you respond? When you're feeling guilty, try to trace where it's coming from. Is it an expectation you've imposed on yourself? Is it realistic? Who are you hoping to appease? Sometimes the expectation is completely unrealistic, and you've set yourself up for both failure and guilt. You might need a friend or professional to help you assess your ability and resources to meet your loved one's needs. Since most caregivers have other responsibilities, such as family and jobs, they are bound to fall short on doing it all. Or they may have their own health issues to address.

Mona's Story

I met several women when my mother was at the rehabilitation center for her broken leg, and I was struck by how two of them desperately wanted to get back home to help take care of their husbands who had health problems. Mona had fractured her femur and was progressing enough to go back home, although the physical therapists felt she could use another week. She had told my mom that she was feeling guilty about leaving Ralph at home and decided to leave early. The first day she returned home, she tripped while assisting him and broke her hip.

In many instances, guilt becomes part of the caregiver equation. The goal is to keep it in check and not let others make you feel guilty for not doing enough when, indeed, you're doing the best you can. Accept that you're human and can't be all things to all people. Sometimes you'll need to set your standards to "real" rather than "ideal" because you simply won't be able to make everything perfect. Letting guilt be the motivating factor in your caregiving is a toxic emotion, so as soon as you hear a guilt-tripping voice in your head, give it a quick listen and, if there's no truth to it, shut it out. Be sure to read the "Caregiver Covenant" section at the end of this chapter to keep feelings of guilt at bay.

Worry

What's going on? Of course, you've got plenty to worry about, and many worries stem from safety concerns—Will your loved one fall, wander off in the haze of Alzheimer's, be alone if he or she has a stroke, or mix up or overdose on medications? Is the cancer progressing, or does he or she have cancer in the first place? These thoughts can make you anxious and interrupt your sleep as your mind keeps racing even though your body desperately wants to shut down. Another underlying emotion that feeds into worry is fear of the future. When will Dad forget who I am? Will we have enough money to keep Mom at home or pay her health-care bills? Will I lose my job if I keep taking off work to drive Mom to dialysis? How will the disease progress?

How should you respond? You're going to worry, and you have cause to do so. But when worry turns into an obsession and has you paralyzed like a deer caught in the headlights or your mind races faster than Mario Andretti, you've got to break the cycle. One solution is to find ways to gain control of what you're worried about. For example, if you're worried about your father's medical prognosis, talk with his physician and ask the questions on your mind. Instead of guessing what can go wrong, acquire accurate details to keep your imagination in check.

Some experts recommend that, instead of spending energy trying to distract yourself from worrying, it's better to set aside some time each day to worry. Carve out 20 minutes to worry; of course, don't do this before you go to bed. If a thought comes up during the day, jot it down and save it for your worry period.

By postponing your worry, you aren't denying it, but you are preventing it from taking over the present. Slowly, you'll gain control of your anxiety. For example, you can share the list of worries that center on caregiving tasks with family members and others who could pick up some of the load.

People who worry tend to focus on "what if," and that leads to identifying a host of problems that they might never even have to solve. So ask yourself whether the problem you are worrying about is something you are facing right now or whether it's a response to a "what if." For example, what if Dad forgets to take his heart medication (even though he never has)? Brainstorm your worries with a problem-solving session to help you sort out what requires your attention and what you can let go or assign to someone else.

One of the hardest things for a worrier to do is accept uncertainty. You might think that if you've thought through all the things that can go wrong, you'll be prepared for whatever the future holds. No surprises for you! But when it comes to caring for an older person, his or her health status can change in the blink of an eye. You'll be better prepared and able to cope with aging's uncertainty by being mindful—observe your thoughts when you're feeling anxious, but don't overanalyze or react to them. In time, the anxiety may pass and you can focus on the present.

Sadness and Depression

What's going on? One of the most overlooked health conditions among older people by their physicians is depression. The "Silent Generation" is pretty mum when it comes to talking about their feelings. If doctors don't ask, parents don't tell. If either of your parents is a caregiver, he or she might not express feeling sadness to you or the doctor. And the general public, including far too many physicians, think that it's normal to be depressed when you're older: just look at all the losses older people have to endure. Many quietly think, "I'd be depressed, too."

If you're a caregiver, you might not realize how depressed and sad you feel because you, too, believe it just goes with the territory. But you should also be aware that you might actually be grieving. It's an emotion we reserve for dying and death, but many caregivers anticipate the loss of loved ones long before they die as they watch them suffer losses, struggle with frailty and pain, and mourn the loss of time spent together as in healthier days. Those contending with Alzheimer's disease know all too well the feeling of "perpetual mourning."

How should you respond? Don't deny your feelings of sadness or feel guilty that you find yourself mourning your loved ones while they are still alive. You'll go through the stages of loss if your parent's condition faces a downward spiral. It will be normal for you to feel emotions of denial, anger, and the litany of "if onlys," "should haves," and "could haves." But if you find yourself feeling so sad that it's affecting your family life, your work, and your ability to care for your parents, you might be experiencing clinical depression—and that needs to be treated by a physician. If not, you'll place yourself at serious risk of compromising your own health.

Resentment

What's going on? Caregivers are notorious for saying "I'd rather do it myself" and believing they're the only ones who can provide the "right" care for their loved ones. The person receiving the care often feeds into this belief because he or she feels more comfortable with the routine they both have established. Other family members are happy to assume that everything is under control and that Mom or Dad likes things just the way they are—and so does Sis. So everything's good. That's one side of the equation.

On the other side is the caregiver sibling or spouse who feels taken for granted and unappreciated. The caregiver resents the lack of help from other family members who don't understand how much the caregiver is going through or the sacrifices the caregiver must make in his or her daily life and at work to care for a loved one. The caregiver begrudges the fact that others don't simply offer to help; he or she resents asking and so doesn't ask. Even though caregivers want to provide the care and are willing to make the sacrifice, they may find that the level of expectations from their care receivers and demand for care is higher than they imagined. They may resent the commitment they now find themselves bound to. They also may be providing care for a difficult parent with whom they have a poor history—perhaps alcoholism or another addiction plagued their childhood. But because of social mores, they feel obligated to help, despite the continued abuse from their parent.

How should you respond? Open up. If you don't express what you're feeling, all this resentment will only turn on you. Your good intentions and compassion in caring for your loved one may turn sour. There is a certain joy to caregiving, and resentment will rob you of it.

Alert

Two other harmful emotional responses that are possible: frustration and isolation. Resentment increases the likelihood that you'll feel alone and that the tasks of daily caregiving will increasingly frustrate you. You'll also become defensive from any advice other family members might offer; through the lens of resentment, you'll interpret it as criticism.

Go back to Chapter 3 and fill out the Caregiving Task Assessment and Caregiving Resource Assessment Worksheets. Share them with family members, and let them know you need and want their participation. Share the worksheets with your parent and ask him or her to help you find solutions to identify more resources—this might include bringing in hired help or volunteers.

Spend some time reflecting on what bothers you most when you're feeling resentful. Is it feeling unappreciated? Do you feel lonely and that you have no one to turn to when you're feeling this way? Is there some pattern to your reaction? Resentment and anger often go hand in hand, so take a look at the strategies for dealing with anger in the next section.

Anger

What's going on? Anger is a completely normal emotion, and in many instances, it can be a healthy reaction to situations that require you to respond assertively to stand up for yourself. When it comes to caregiving, anger is an emotion that you can manage. You can control it, and you "own" it. Even when you feel that your mom or dad makes you angry, the truth is, no one can *make* you angry. *You* make yourself angry. Sure, something your parent does can provoke you, but you get to decide how you're going to respond to that provocation.

To better understand what provokes you, break your anger into small parts. Think about the last three or four times you became angry with your parent. Can you recall what you were feeling *before* you saw Mom or Dad? Were you feeling pulled in too many directions? Were you squeezing in your visit between other family responsibilities?

Now think about what your parent said or did that displeased you. Was it something about the tone of voice? Did you feel the request was given as an order? Is your parent not doing what you asked? What action did you need to do just before you got angry—was it cleaning up after him or her? Getting Mom or Dad in and out of the car and dealing with parking after a hassle through traffic? Do you see any kind of pattern in a certain activity or certain behaviors that "push your button"? Could any of this be related to old, unresolved issues with your parent?

What did you physically feel when you got angry? Was your heart racing, your stomach in knots, your face flushed, your teeth clenched, or your head pounding? Anger triggers physical reactions that cause your heart rate and blood pressure to go up, and it affects the energy level of your hormones. When you've identified these components to your anger, you can start developing a plan of action to take control of each.

How should you respond? Communication is key to healthy expressions of anger. Dr. Stephen F. Duncan, professor of the School of Family Life at Bringham Young University, suggests that the best way to express anger is to use "I-statements with a Feeling-When-Because format."

Here's an example: "Mom, *I feel* upset *when* I've taken off work to drive you to the doctor's *because* what I've done for you isn't acknowledged. *I* feel unappreciated." Notice these are all statements that tell her how you're feeling instead of accusing her of being ungrateful. Who knows? She may be feeling resentful that she has to depend on you and can't get past her own anger to appreciate what you're doing. Or maybe she's embarrassed about needing your help. Use this as an opportunity to try to understand what's behind her actions that provoke you.

Find ways that are calming to you as soon as you feel the physical signs of anger; it might be leaving the room and taking a deep breath, taking a short walk, envisioning a scene that's peaceful, or calling a friend. When it comes to sharing your feelings, speak slowly and lower your voice, and sit down next to your mom or dad in a manner that shows you want to solve this problem. This isn't about denying your anger; it's about *listening* to it instead of letting it toss you into a sea of seething.

Everyday Stress Relievers

If you've learned anything from this chapter, hopefully it is that caregiving—no matter how good you feel about it or how well intentioned you are—is stressful. And it's stressful not every so often, but nearly every day. Here's a list of stress relievers you can use on a daily basis:

- Reserve 10 to 15 minutes a day to yourself. Most caregivers think they have no time and scoff at advice to put aside time for themselves. If you can, make it the same time, and earlier in the day, before "life" gets in the way. Listen to music, have a quiet cup of tea, sit in front of a window to enjoy the sun, or just do something nurturing.

- Find a way to get some exercise—take the stairs more often, walk at a brisk pace around the house, or hold a dance party with yourself. Just a few minutes jumping around to your favorite tunes can do wonders in releasing those oxytocin hormones we talked about. Ask a friend or neighbor to spend 15 minutes with your loved one so you can go outside and take a walk. Give yoga a try—watch it on television or get a DVD.

- Breathe. Deep breaths and breathing exercises throughout the day do a body good, as does drinking frequent glasses of fresh water. Envision something soothing while you're at it.

- Connect with your friends, support groups, or church or synagogue. When you need to vent, instead of holding it in, share it with someone who can listen and help you calmly get through it.

- Get yourself a batch of small index cards and write on each one a small task that you would be more than happy to have someone do. It could be spending time with your parent so you can take a walk, pick up medications at the pharmacy, drop off or make dinner, visit for lunch, accompany you on a doctor's visit so parking won't be such a hassle, or pick up groceries. When someone says to you, "Is there anything I can do?" appreciatively say yes and let him or her choose a card.

- If past grievances and conflicts with family members keep getting in the way, or if you ever strike out in anger, seek professional advice.

- Place inspirational quotes or reminders on your mirror. Remind yourself to take one day at a time, remember that you're doing the best you can, focus on your loved one's abilities instead of limitations, and look for the humor in the day. Laugh, and then laugh some more.

- Confess. Hold your own personal confession and then forgive yourself. You're going to make mistakes, and chances are, you'll regret things that you've said. Admit them, apologize, and create a solution for the next time. My guess is that even Mother Theresa had her moments.

Humor: It's There If You Look for It

When I was caring for Lena (my husband's grandmother), she was going through a stage of paranoia and one morning told me she was getting ready to go see the police. I asked her why. She told me that I was poisoning her. My husband quipped, "No, Grandma, that's just how Linda cooks—you'll get used to it." That seemed to satisfy her, and we all just broke down and laughed. It also helped me laugh off some of the stress I was feeling that day.

Respite Care by the Day and Vacations

If you're taking care of a loved one with dementia or someone who has physical or communication difficulties that are quite demanding, look for respite care programs in your community. Most of them are spelled out in Chapter 6. Adult day services should be at the top of your list, because they not only give you a much-needed break, but they also help your loved one function and feel better. Even just three half-days a week will make a significant difference in the quality of your life and theirs.

Taking vacations, or at least enjoying a long weekend away, is one of the first casualties of caregiving. But at some point, everyone needs to take time off to recharge. One way of managing a getaway is to set up a "mutual vacation" in which your parent takes a "vacation" at a quality assisted living facility while you and your husband or friend go out of town. Many assisted living facilities are delighted to have a short-stay guest, often referred to as "respite care." Your parent may actually enjoy all the attention and dining out every day, along with the security of having his or her physical needs met.

Just make sure that this option is okay with your parent and that you both visit the facility ahead of time, perhaps to have lunch or dinner together. Your parent should not feel like she is being abandoned or set up for eventual placement in what she may consider a nursing home. Most facilities require a refundable deposit, depending on the length of stay.

The following is a lovely letter from one of my readers, who described how he and his wife arranged a mutual vacation for his mother, who lived with them. This amazing couple provides a good example of how thoughtful planning can allow you to enjoy a guilt-free vacation while your loved one is safely being cared for.

We personally visited several retirement communities, and eliminated some on sight and others because they did not provide the flexibility we needed. The one we ultimately chose had neither a minimum nor a maximum period for so-called "respite" care. We planned our loved one's vacation so that she entered the facility a day or two before we left town, and it extended two or three days on the other end. That way, if adjustment problems arose or medication problems surfaced (that happens!), we would be around to see to the problem. At the other end of the vacation period, we had a couple of days to unpack and "re-enter" without coping with caregiving needs. During the vacation period, we made arrangements for drop-in visits by friends of the family.

We also planned the mailing of cards so that the week was pretty much covered by mail each day. We arranged for the newspaper to be delivered to her so that she had her own paper for crossword puzzles. We arranged with a local florist to have a fresh arrangement sent at the midpoint to cheer up the room and remind her that we were thinking of her. (For a man, some florists will make up and deliver "snack baskets" with little boxes and bags of this and that.) As

continues

continued

a bonus, when the time came for her to enter assisted living full time, she related to her very pleasant "vacations" rather than feeling threatened or, at worst, abandoned.

If your loved one does not need 'round-the-clock care, you might want to consider bringing in someone from a nonmedical senior care agency for a weekend or ask a family member or friend to stay.

Support Groups: Real and Virtual

One way of dealing with the stress of caregiving is to share your feelings and experiences with others who are going through the same thing. As the famous British writer Dorothy L. Sayers wrote, "Trouble shared is trouble halved." I've always been inspired by the resourcefulness of family caregivers, especially when they share their own tips on how to make the job easier or how they've learned to cope. Hearing it from others who know the "real deal" resonates so much more than being told what you should do from well-meaning friends who have no idea what life is really like for you.

You can find support groups by calling your local hospital, senior center, or adult day center. If your loved one has dementia, be sure to call your local Alzheimer's chapter. If your loved one has a health condition such as cancer, heart disease, or Parkinson's, go to national websites to find local chapters or find them in the Yellow Pages. Most disease-based organizations offer support groups, and some offer online support groups as well.

If you can't get out to support group meetings (but please do try), go online to join a chat group or blog, or just read through comments made by other caregivers. One such site is www.caring.com, where you'll find articles from experts, blogs, guides, checklists, and directories of long-term care services nationwide. If you're caring for a loved one with Alzheimer's, join the Steps and Stages support groups. Another helpful feature is "Caregiver Confessions," by Leeza Gibbons.

You can also organize your own inner circle of family and friends, and email each other or create a private Facebook page to share ideas, thoughts, and feelings. And then there's the phone. You can actually talk to people. What is the message? Reach out and let others in.

Caregiver Covenant

I've developed a Caregiver Covenant to guide you along your caregiving journey. You can download a printed version at www.lindarhodescaregiving.com under "Caregiver Tips."

To the best of my ability, I will …

- Solicit the preferences and values of my loved one so I can provide and arrange for care that respects their person and is centered upon meeting their needs and wishes.

- Advocate for my loved one by educating myself on caregiving matters—health conditions, care plans, and medications—so I can ask informed questions and better monitor their care.

- Research the quality of care services, facilities, and persons who provide care to my loved one to ensure their well-being.

- Support my loved one's desire for independence and dignity while addressing their need to remain safe and secure.

- Foster a caregiving relationship that espouses mutual trust, respect, kindness, and patience while disavowing behavior that evokes feelings of guilt or resentment.

- Reach out for and accept help from family, friends, community, and volunteers, recognizing that caregiving as a solo act is not healthy for my loved one or for me.

- Nurture my body, mind, and spirit by taking the time to care for myself, replenish my soul, and seek respite from my caregiving.

- Forgive and learn from my shortcomings realizing that I'm only human and will have my moments of feeling frustrated, angry, or sad. If these feelings dominate my caregiving, I'll seek professional help.

- Preserve my family and professional life throughout my caregiving in a manner that will not jeopardize or harm what I hold dear.

- Cherish the purpose, bond, and meaning that caring for my loved one brings to my life and make room for the healing power of humor and laughter.

Many before you have traveled this path. May you follow in their footsteps with wisdom and grace.

Essential Takeaways

- Caregivers experience joyful moments and feelings, but they also experience stress—and sometimes a great deal of it. Ignoring the telltale signs of too much stress can be dangerous.

- Learn to break down what you're feeling so you can identify the underlying emotions that fuel them and make adjustments when needed.

- You actually do have time for yourself, and it's up to you to take control.

- Reach out, let others in, and share the load.

Part 2

The Elder Care Landscape: Know More, Act Confidently

The field of elder care has mushroomed over the last decade in response to the aging tsunami throughout the country. Search for "elder care" or "caregiving" on the World Wide Web, and you're in for millions of "hits" on living options, resources, products, health-care services, and a never-ending stream of information on age-related diseases and conditions. It's easy to get lost.

If you understand the elder care landscape, you'll navigate it well and reach destinations that make the most sense for your mother or father. Your parent's health and caregiving needs are a work in progress, and so, too, must be your responses.

Identify the foremost caregiving services and help lines you'll want at your fingertips. Learn what each offers and the savvy questions to ask as you explore them. Today your parents have a wide range of living arrangements from which to choose; find out what they are, how to access reports that rate their quality, what to look for on a site visit, and factors to consider in making the best choice for your parent's needs.

Legal issues abound in the world of elder care. Learn how to discuss wills, durable health-care power of attorney, and advance directives. Gain a better understanding of what "do not resuscitate" orders mean and why guardianship should be used only as a last resort.

chapter 6

Caregiving Services to the Rescue

Working with geriatric care managers

Community services and public resources around you

Adult day centers for a parent with dementia

Professional health-care services for home

The benefits of nonmedical senior care

I know it's hard to steal away the time to look for help and make calls when you're in the throes of caregiving, but an hour here and there doing a bit of research can make a huge difference in the lives of you and your loved one. It really is worth the treasure hunt. So instead of turning this into a frantic scavenger hunt like the hit show *The Amazing Race,* I've found the answers for you. All you have to do is make the calls.

Geriatric Care Managers

Juggling long-distance caregiving, getting professional advice on how to organize your parent's care, and figuring out what your parent needs just got easier with the emergence of geriatric care managers (GCMs). This is a relatively new profession of social workers, counselors, and nurses who assess, organize, monitor, and manage your parent's caregiving needs. GCMs are also referred to as Elder Care Managers or Care Coordinators.

The GCM's first step is usually to meet with you and your parent for an initial conference, to identify everyone's needs. The GCM can also arrange for a comprehensive geriatric assessment that brings together an interdisciplinary team to holistically examine your loved one (see Chapter 1), or the GCM might conduct an independent assessment. When you have a solid understanding of your parent's health and functional status, then you, your parent, and the GCM can realistically and knowledgeably craft a viable care plan. Based on the plan, you can decide which part the GCM will perform and what you and other family members will handle.

A GCM can provide a wide array of services, including:

- Determine eligibility for a host of services; make arrangements for those services

- Interview home health-care and personal care workers and monitor their performance

- Arrange for transportation to and from doctor's appointments; accompany patients to appointments and report back to family members

- Analyze financial, legal, and medical information

- Pay bills

- Find a quality rehabilitation center, assisted living facility, or skilled nursing facility

- Oversee the transition from hospital discharge to home

- Manage a move from your parent's home

GCMs charge for their services in a variety of ways. Depending on what services you agree upon, you might be charged hourly, weekly, or monthly rates or you might pay for a package of services. Fees range from $100 to $200 per hour, depending on the care manager's credentials, experience, and local economies. Out-of-pocket expenses commonly cover mileage, caregiving supplies, and services of additional consultants or health-care providers that you've requested.

The initial assessment might cost $250 or more; based upon your parent's needs, you and the GCM then agree on a care plan. Make sure all of this is entered in writing and that you have clear expectations of what services will be performed. Keep in mind, though, that these services can also save money in the long term: A GCM has expertise in securing benefits and ensuring that the most appropriate level of care is provided to your parent, preventing premature deterioration that could eventually require very expensive nursing home care.

Medicare does not cover GCM services; a long-term care insurance policy might cover them, but most often, this is a private-pay, out-of-pocket expense.

When you interview a GCM, here's what to ask:

- What services do you offer and who actually provides them?

- What are your credentials? Are you licensed in your profession?

- How long have you been providing care-management services? How long have you been practicing in this community?

- Do you have any affiliations and memberships in community organizations?

- Are you available for emergencies? Who is your backup if you are not available?

- What can I expect to learn from your initial assessment? What does it include (for example, physical and mental status, financial resources)?

- Who conducts the medical component of the assessment, and what are his or her qualifications? Do I pay for this separately? Will Medicare cover any of this expense?

- How do you perform quality checks on the service providers and referrals you recommend?

- How do you communicate information to me about my parent, and how often do you do so?

- How often will you have face-to-face contact with my parent?

- How many cases do you handle at one time?

- What are your fees, and can you provide me with references?

It's vital that you do your homework by verifying the GCM's credentials. Currently, this profession is essentially an unregulated field because anyone can open a practice and claim to be a GCM. Be sure to ask whether the GCM has received any type of certification, where it is from, and whether he or she is a member of the National Association of Professional GCMs. Just be aware, however, that this is a nonprofit association, not a credentialing institution.

Tip

To find a geriatric care manager, call the National Association of Professional Geriatric Care Managers at 520-881-8008 or visit the website at www. caremanager.org. On the site, go to "Find a Care Manager," where you can search by state and zip code for a local GCM and a description of the services offered and the degree he or she holds. You will also find GCMs listed in the Yellow Pages, under "Social Workers," "Elder Care," and/or "Home Health Care."

If your parent has a low or moderate income, he or she might qualify for care-management services similar to what GCMs offer privately through the local Area Agency on Aging (AAA). Find your local agency by calling the Eldercare Locator at 1-800-677-1116, or go to www.eldercare.gov, and ask about the Community Waiver or Options program.

Community Services

When you start doing your research, you might find a wealth of community services right around the corner. You might be surprised at the variety of ways community groups and agencies are marshaling their efforts to help caregivers care for their loved ones. Check out the following chart for possible services in your area.

Community Services in a Nutshell

Kind of Service	What It Is	Find It
Information and referral	Experts identify what you need and where to find it.	Senior centers, Area Agencies on Aging (AAA), hospitals. Call 211 or visit www.211.org.
Home-delivered meals	"Meals on Wheels" are delivered to homebound elderly.	Senior centers, churches, synagogues, AAA, National Meals on Wheels (1-800-999-6262).
Telephone reassurance	Volunteers make daily calls to make sure the elder is okay.	Senior centers, AAA, hospital volunteers.
Chore services	Volunteers make minor repairs to the home and perform handyman services.	AAA, weatherization programs, Supportive Housing & Home Modifications Foundation. Call: 213-740-1364 or visit www.homemods.org.
Transportation	Drivers provide free and reduced rides to senior centers, clinics, day centers, and shopping areas.	"Shared ride" programs via AAA, senior centers, public transit authority.
Respite care	Volunteers give caregivers a break by caring for their elders.	AAA, senior centers, faith-based groups. For a fee, nursing homes and assisted living centers provide weekend care and more.
Friendly visitor companion program	Volunteers visit, run errands, and provide companionship.	Senior centers, faith-based groups, AAA, Corporation for National Service (1-800-424-8867), local high school service projects.

Kind of Service	What It Is	Find It
Senior centers	Volunteers offer meals, social recreational activities, health screens, and educational activities.	Phone book under "Senior Centers," AAA, Eldercare Locator (1-800-677-1116).
Legal services, elder protective services, ombudsman	Experts offer help with financial and legal problems, report suspected abuse or neglect, and help with complaints against LTC facilities.	AAA, Legal Services listed in the Blue Pages, AARP Legal Helpline (1-800-772-1213).
Free health screenings, flu shots, support groups	Elders receive free health screenings, immunizations, tests, and emotional support.	Hospitals, pharmacies, events at local malls. Get on your local hospital's community newsletter mailing list.
Grocery and medication delivery	Medications and groceries are sent to your elder.	Pharmacies, grocery stores, volunteer groups.
Volunteer service projects	A wide range of services are performed for the elderly living at home or in a long-term care facility.	Local service clubs such as Rotary, Lions, and Zonta; Catholic Charities and Jewish Family Services, and other religious groups.

Adult Day Centers

I've spent several years as president of a volunteer board of directors for an adult day center. It's been an inspiring tenure witnessing families who heroically care for their loved ones so they can remain at home rather than be placed in a facility. Some people drop off a parent early in the morning while they go onto work and then return home for a "second shift."

Other family members are older spouses who use the time to regroup or run errands because it's not safe to leave their husband or wife home alone. Whether working or needing respite care, all the families are grateful for what the center has done for their loved one: "Mom just beams when she comes here." "Dad is like a new person." "Without this place, my wife would be in a nursing home." If there's one message our families would tell you, it is that they wish they had pursued this service sooner. It helped their loved one better function, and it helped them provide better care.

If you have a loved one who has physical disabilities, cognitive difficulties (thinking), or dementia, or requires assistance with the tasks of daily living and is not able to remain safely alone, absolutely consider adult day services.

Centers offer activities that help participants maintain memory and function through therapeutic activities, music therapy, socialization, nutritious meals, speech therapy, physical exercises, brain fitness exercises, physical therapy, and nursing care.

All that mental stimulation and physical activity improves their sleep, which many a caregiver recognizes as a godsend. The goal of adult day centers is to foster well-being, enhance functioning, and promote health for their participants.

Basically three types of adult day centers exist: social models that cater to higher-functioning participants, health-centered models that provide nursing care, and Alzheimer's/dementia care centers. The latter two models are often combined. Families use adult day centers to gain respite from caregiving, especially for older spouses who care for a loved one with dementia, or to maintain a job while their family member lives with them.

Adult day centers often operate from about 7:00 A.M. to 6:00 P.M. to accommodate the schedules of working caregivers, and many are open up to seven days a week. You can expect to pay the national average of $67 per day or less if it is purely a social model, or more if nursing care is also provided.

Medicare does not cover adult day services; however, Medicaid (state-funded long-term care) might pay for it, if you meet certain income limits and the service prevents nursing home placement. To see whether you qualify, call the Eldercare Locator at 1-800-677-1116 to find your local Area Agency on Aging. The Veterans Administration also assists families in paying for adult day services for veterans who qualify. Many long-term care insurance policies cover the service.

You can find a local adult day center by looking in the Yellow Pages under "Adult Day Care," "Adult Day Services," or "Aging Service." An online search using key words "adult day center" or "adult day services" should quickly generate a list of centers in your area. You can also find centers by visiting the National Adult Day Services Association's website at www.nadsa.org or calling 1-877-745-1440.

When you call a center, the National Adult Day Services Association suggests that you ask these questions:

- Who owns or sponsors the agency?

- How long has it been operating? (The longer, the better.)

- What is your licensure status? (Ask for the name of the licensing agency and a copy of the current license.)

- How can I review reports of surveyors who inspect your facility?

- What are the days and hours of operation?

- Is transportation to and from the center provided?

- Which conditions are accepted (for example, memory loss, limited mobility, and incontinence)?

- What are the staff's credentials and background checks, and what is the ratio of staff to participants?

- What type of ongoing training do you offer to your staff?

- What type of programming do you offer for dementia clients?

- What safety features do you provide so that clients don't wander from the premises?

- What activities are offered? Are there a variety of individual and group programs?

- Are meals and snacks included? Are special diets accommodated?

- How do you let the caregivers know how well their loved one is doing at the center?

- Do you perform a health-care assessment or require one before my loved one attends?

- What are your rates, and what do you charge for additional services?

Spend a day at the center(s) to get a sense of the people attending, the staff, and the environment to determine whether it is the best fit for your parent. You might need to convince your loved one that he or she is going to a meeting or some favorite activity. The social worker at the center should be helpful in identifying ways to help your parent feel comfortable during those first few transitional days.

Home Health Care

As the term implies, home health care provides health-care services in the home, initiated by a required prescription from a physician. If your parent needs nursing care or care provided by another licensed professional, such as a physical, respiratory, or occupational therapist, you should approach a home health-care agency for the care.

Let's say your mom is recovering from a hip fracture. The hospital or rehab facility is discharging her to go home, but she still needs physical therapy and a nurse to care for a wound she developed from the fall. In this case, a physician would write a prescription for her care, and she would choose a home health-care agency to provide the therapy and nursing service. The home health agency would send a nurse to your mother's home to assess her needs and develop a care plan to treat her as ordered by her doctor.

A social worker or discharge planner at the hospital likely will provide you with a packet of information on home health care that includes a list of Medicare-certified agencies. Look for agencies that are Medicare certified so that, if your parent meets certain conditions, Medicare will cover some or all of her care for a designated period of time. Medicare certification also means that the agency has met federal minimum requirements for patient care and management; as a result, it can charge Medicare and Medicaid (state welfare) for services rendered.

A home health-care agency employs the health-care professionals being sent to your home; it is state licensed, and many seek accreditation to assure consumers that they have met the high quality standards of their industry. Two common accreditations you might recognize are Accreditation Commission for Health Care (ACHC) and Joint Commission on Accreditation of Healthcare Organizations (JCAHO).

Be aware that home health-care "registries" do not employ the caregiver sent to your home. They are employment agencies for home health-care workers. Thus, you are responsible for paying the worker's taxes and following health and labor laws. Be sure to find out whether the agency you use actually employs the workers or is merely a registry.

Medicare does not cover all forms of home health care, so ask what's covered (or not), given your parent's circumstances, when you conduct interviews. These agencies can be freestanding, such as the VNA, or a hospital might operate its own agency. You can find them online or in the phone book under "Home Health" or "Home Health Care Agency."

When searching for a home health-care agency, here are questions to ask:

- Are you Medicare certified? If so, Medicare will reimburse the agency for services performed.

- Do you offer the services the doctor has prescribed? Will any personal care services be provided (for example, help with bathing, dressing, and transferring), and will this be covered?

- Do you have accreditations from professional organizations? If so, what are they?

- What type of background checks do you conduct on all your employees?

- Are these individuals your full-time employees?

- If someone does not show up to care for my loved one, will you send a replacement immediately?

- What type of reports can I expect on my loved one's progress from each type of professional treating him or her?

- What is your state licensure status?

- Will you send a replacement care provider if the initial provider doesn't work well with my loved one?

- What can I expect to pay out of pocket for services not covered by my loved one's insurance (for example, Medicare, Medigap, Medicaid, or long-term care insurance policy)?

- Who do I speak to regarding my loved one's status? Is this the same person coordinating his or her care or providing it?

- How do I appeal to Medicare if we think more care is needed?

- Are you handling the claims to Medicare? Or do we have to pay first and then are reimbursed by Medicare?

- Could you please provide me with letters and references from other families who have used your service?

- Is staff available on weekends and in emergencies?

One of the best ways to determine whether the agency offers quality care is to use Medicare's "Compare Home Health Agencies" tool found on its home page at www.medicare.gov. Just by entering your parent's zip code, you can find the name and contact information of local home health agencies, the services each agency offers, whether the agency is Medicare certified, and its type of ownership (for example, for-profit versus non-profit). After you choose the agencies that offer the services your parent needs, you can simply click each one and find out how each compares on 12 quality measures. You'll even learn how the agency's ratings stack up against other home health-care agencies in the state and the nation.

You'll learn the percentage of patients who have less pain when moving around, who get better at taking their medicines, whose bladder control improves, and whose wounds improve and heal after surgery. You'll also see the percentage of patients who are readmitted to a hospital; who need urgent, unplanned care; or who have wounds that have gotten worse or developed under the agency's care.

If you don't have internet service, call Medicare at 1-800-633-4227 and ask whether it'll give you quality measure information on home health-care agencies that you are considering. Also ask for a free copy of *Medicare and Home Health Care,* an excellent guide for consumers that describes what you need to know in finding and utilizing home health care. You can also download a copy at its website.

By using the "Compare Home Health Agencies" tool and asking the right questions, you'll be in good shape to find your parent an agency that will take good care of him or her for a smooth and speedy recovery.

Nonmedical Senior Care

Senior care, home care, and nonmedical senior care companies offer personalized assistance with the tasks of daily living for older people at home. I call it "stitch in time" care because it enables people to remain independent, socially engaged, and still at home. Companies offering senior care make it clear that they provide *nonmedical* services. In other words, they are not in the home health-care business or offering nursing care.

Instead, they offer companionship, meal preparation, medication reminders, light housework, transportation, errands, grocery shopping, pharmacy pickups, appointment arrangement, bill and letter mailing, and a stable bathing environment, to name a few.

If you're worried that your dad isn't getting enough social interaction, this type of company can match him up with someone he enjoys spending time with engaging in his favorite hobbies, movies, or games, or good conversation.

There's been an explosion in the senior care industry over the last several years. You'll find senior care companies listed in the phone book under "Home Care." Some are franchises, as with Home Instead Senior Care, Wisdom Keepers, Comfort Care, Visiting Angels, and Comfort Keepers; others are independently owned. Home Instead Senior Care is an international franchise that offers advanced training in Alzheimer's for its caregivers.

Alert

In many states, these companies are not licensed by a state agency because they offer nonmedical care. So that means, as a consumer, you need to do your research.

Here's a list of questions that can help you identify the best agency for your parent:

- Do you conduct criminal background checks on your employees, and are they bonded?

- Are the caregivers your employees, or are you a registry (meaning you are paying taxes and Social Security)?

- What type of training do your employees go through to be hired? What ongoing training do they receive?

- Have your caregivers been trained in how to properly lift and help transfer a patient?

- Please describe the background of your average caregiver (for example, part-time homemaker, certified nurse's aide, high school graduate, or retiree).

- What kind of progress reports and care notes can I expect to receive on my parent's care? Who do I speak to if I have any questions or need to update you on my parent's needs?

- If you provide transportation, have you verified and reviewed your employee's driving record?

- How do you ensure that the caregiver is compatible with my parent?

- How long have most of your employees worked for you?

- Are your services covered by long-term care insurance, and will you process the paperwork?

- How do you supervise and oversee the quality of care your workers provide?

- May I see a sample service agreement and a listing of your prices? Is a minimum number of hours required for each visit?

In terms of additional background research, check to see whether any complaints have been lodged against the company through the Better Business Bureau. Call the *ombudsman* of your local Area Agency on Aging to see whether he or she knows of any complaints against the company (call Eldercare Locator at 1-800-677-1116 to find your local Area Agency on Aging). I'd also ask whether the agency will allow you to speak with customers who have used the service.

Ombudsman is a Swedish term meaning "representative." The ombudsman's job is to help solve problems among residents, their families, and the staff in long-term care facilities. Every nursing home is assigned an ombudsman, who is usually an employee of the local Area Agency on Aging.

You'll find that prices range from $12 to $22 per hour, depending on local economies; there's usually a minimum service requirement of at least two hours. Services can be arranged for as many as 24 hours a day for a short-term or long-term arrangement, including weekends and holidays. This can be especially helpful when families need respite from daily caregiving.

Some long-term care insurance policies do cover nonmedical senior care, so be sure to look over your parent's policy, if she has one.

You might also find volunteer senior-care services provided by faith-based organizations, so if you are financially strapped, give your local church or synagogue a call to see what it provides. Local senior centers might also be a good resource for finding nonprofit groups that offer volunteer senior care. The national Family Caregiver Support Program funded through Area Agencies on Aging might also be a resource for you, if you qualify. You learn more about this opportunity in the next section.

Public Caregiving Programs

Enter the term "elder care" in your internet browser search bar, and within seconds, Google will spew out a volcanic 50 million responses. Enter "public caregiving programs," and a mere 7 million responses pop up. Even if you look over just the first 10 pages of entries, it's beyond overwhelming.

Let me make it easier for you and narrow the list to six core public benefit programs and resources that can assist you in your caregiving. You'll also find a Resource Directory in Appendix A that reviews some of the leading programs and services. If you go to my website at www. lindarhodescaregiving.com, you'll find all the websites hyperlinked for you. Just go to the Resources navigation bar.

Eldercare Locator: Locating Services Nationwide

If you're looking for elder care services and resources in your community or state, or any state throughout the country, this site is a one-stop shop. It is administered by the federal Administration on Aging. Throughout this book, I remind you to call the Eldercare Locator's toll-free number at 1-800-677-1116 as a quick reference for tracking down the service or program being discussed. Or you can go to its website at www.eldercare.gov and view the Quick Index so you can easily link to all the services offered by the Administration on Aging. You can find the Area Agency on Aging closest to your parent and access other caregiving websites as well.

Area Agencies on Aging

Every community throughout the country has access to an Area Agency on Aging (AAA). Funded by the federal Older American's Act and state funds, these agencies are the central planners, organizers, and care managers of aging services within your county. They are also your community's chief advocate on issues facing older people.

Area Agencies on Aging act as a major provider and subcontractor of aging services devoted to giving older adults the option to live at home and remain in their communities. The agency funds senior centers, home-delivered meals, and shared-ride programs, and it serves as the state's watchdog in protecting vulnerable elders by implementing protective service laws and operating ombudsman programs in long-term care facilities.

The following are three of the major ways you can take advantage of your local AAA:

- **Information hub.** Because the agency is responsible for planning aging services for the whole community, it knows just about every program in the region. Many agencies offer guidebooks of all the services available. You can track down your local Area Agency on

Aging's website by going to www.eldercare.gov. Just enter your parent's county and click "General Information and Assistance" on the search bar. The local AAA can tell you what services are available, advise you on eligibility criteria of various programs, and provide contact information. Or just call the Eldercare Locator, at 1-800-677-1116, to find the closest agency to your parent. You can also find it listed in the Blue Pages of your phone book.

- **Care management.** If your parent has a modest income, he or she might qualify for a caseworker and a team of professionals skilled in geriatric social work and nursing to help manage their care. They'll assess your parent's needs and bring together the services required to take care of your parent and help him or her remain in the community. For example, they might arrange for adult day services for a loved one with dementia while the caregiver is at work, send in-home delivered meals, and arrange for a caregiver to come in three times a week and to provide a weekly nursing assessment. Each plan is tailored to an individual's needs. The AAA also provides geriatric assessments to determine whether your parent needs nursing home care or assisted living. Each program has eligibility guidelines, so you need to call to find out if your parent qualifies.

- **Family Caregiver Support Program.** This national program is offered in every state through your local AAA. If you are taking care of a loved one 60 years of age or older who has a moderate income, he or she might qualify. In the AAA, "family caregiver" is defined simply as "an adult family member, or another individual, who is an informal provider of in-home and community care to an older individual." The program operates on a sliding fee scale, so it is not a poverty-restricted program. The age restriction of 60 years is removed if your parent suffers from dementia. Many programs pay $200 a month for out-of-pocket expenses that families spend on services and supplies to maintain a loved one at home. Some programs also offer up to $2,000 in home modifications so that a ramp or stair climb, for example, can be installed. You can also receive a family consultation, legal advice, a needs assessment, respite care, and caregiver education and training. Another component of the program assists grandparents age 55 and up who are acting as primary caregivers for grandchildren or other related children age 18 or under and living in the grandparent's home.

Home and Community-Based Services Waiver Programs

With federal approval, states may waive the use of their Medical Assistance dollars received from the federal government for skilled nursing facility–based care and instead redirect them to a variety of programs that maintain older people in their homes and communities.

Known as Home and Community-Based Services (HCBS) 1915(c) waivers, they allow the provision of long-term care services in home- and community-based settings under the Medicaid Program. These state programs offer lower-income individuals who are ill enough to qualify for nursing home care the opportunity to stay at home by providing them with services such as home care, assistance with daily living tasks, nursing care, care management, respite care, adult day services, and caregiving supplies. Many of these programs are coordinated between the state unit on aging and the state Medical Assistance agency (for example, Department of Public Welfare or Department of Human Services).

So if you have a loved one who needs care that would qualify him or her for skilled nursing home care, but you'd like to receive resources and support to keep him or her at home, the best way to find out what's available is to call your local Area Agency on Aging.

The Veterans Administration

Often people think that if they don't live in a community with a Veterans Affairs Medical Center, they can't receive elder care services. However, if a veteran has been enrolled and accepted, he can receive primary care from outpatient clinics, community-based care, nursing home care, home-based primary care, adult day care, rehabilitation, diagnostic and treatment services, and hospital (medical and surgical) inpatient care. If the VA doesn't operate a facility where your father lives, it can send him to one located nearest him or subcontract with a provider to give him the service. To learn if your father qualifies for enrollment, call 1-877-222-VETS or visit the website at www.va.gov.

The Veterans Administration also provides a VA Caregiver Support program. If a veteran is unable to perform an activity of daily living or needs supervision or protection based on an impairment or injury (such as dementia, stroke, or Parkinson's disease), the caregiver may qualify for up to 30 days of respite care per year, support groups, and education and training on caregiving. The veteran might qualify for a wide range of long-term care services that include home modifications, medical equipment, and vehicle modification. To find out more, go to www.caregiver.va.gov or call the National Caregiver Support Line at 855-260-3274.

Medicare

Medicare is the centerpiece of your parents' health care; we discuss it in greater detail in Chapter 10. What's covered and what's not are always changing, and the best way to keep up with the benefits and eligibility guidelines is to regularly visit the website, at www.medicare.gov, which is extremely well done. If you do not have internet access, you can also call 1-800-MEDICARE (1-800-633-4227).

If your parents are Medicare beneficiaries, take the time to review the annual *Medicare & You Handbook* that's mailed to them every year and describes their benefits and what is covered. You can also access the guide online; it has a nice search function to make finding what you need easier.

The feature I like most is the ratings and comparison reports on nursing homes, home health-care agencies, hospitals, Medigap policies, drug plans, and durable medical goods and equipment companies. For example, if you're looking for a nursing home, you can find the results of the latest inspection report on every nursing home in the country and see how many stars Medicare awarded a facility, according to its five-star rating system. You can compare nursing homes in your area and receive contact information on each.

Medicare also features a "Caregiver Resources" site with information organized from the perspective of what a caregiver might ask, especially in terms of what services are covered. For this customized section of the website, go to www.medicare.gov/caregivers.

Benefits Checkup

This screening service is free from the National Council on Aging. Fill out the online forms and learn whether you qualify for any of the thousands of state, national, and private programs in the database. You can also find out whether your parent qualifies for Extra Help for Medicare Part D, food stamps, and assistance with health care, home care, meals, utility bills, and more. This is a web-based service only, at www.benefitscheckup.org.

You'll be asked to fill out a questionnaire that takes only 10 to 15 minutes to complete. Enter basic information on your parent, including income (all info remains confidential). After you've entered the data, the Benefits Checkup searches thousands of benefits against your parent's information. Within seconds, you'll receive an Eligibility Report that identifies potential benefits for which your parent might be eligible. The report includes the information you need to contact the local agency to determine whether your parent actually qualifies. You will get local names, addresses, and toll-free phone numbers, along with application forms that you simply download and send to the appropriate agency. This resource is a great timesaver!

The Benefits Checkup website is especially helpful if you live in a different state than your parents because it searches thousands of programs by state and gives you local numbers to contact.

Essential Takeaways

- You might feel that you don't have the time to research your options or reach out for help, but the return on investment for you and your loved one is absolutely worth it.
- Eldercare Locator, at 1-800-677-1116, and your local Area Agency on Aging act as your information hub and central point of access for a wide range of community-based long-term care services.

- If you are caring for a loved one who has dementia or struggles with the results of a stroke or Parkinson's disease, consider an adult day center for his or her benefit and yours.

- Eligibility for many elder care public programs does not require poverty-level income. An easy one-stop website to determine your parent's eligibility for thousands of programs is offered at www.benefitscheckup.org.

chapter 7

Finding the Best Living Option for Your Parent

Meeting the challenges of living at home

Fostering independence with senior living communities

Understanding what assisted living centers really offer

What to look for in skilled nursing facilities

Creative living options

In days gone by, the choice of where you lived during life's later years was rather straightforward. You lived mostly at home, or if you became very ill and demanded care beyond what family members could provide, you entered a nursing home. Today there are as many living options as there are cell-phone plans.

Now that people are living longer and coping with an array of chronic conditions, adaptive housing options abound. Add to that the aging of a huge number of baby boomers, and it's easy to explain why senior living choices are exploding.

So let's take a look at the different living options available to your parents and see what makes the most sense, given their circumstances.

Living at Home

Given a choice, 9 out of 10 people want to remain at home for the duration of their lives. This is especially so for a generation that takes great pride in owning a home. Living on their own, whether it's in an apartment or a house, also represents independence and self-reliance—two hallmark traits of the older generation. It's no wonder, then, that even when illness or physical disabilities befall your parents, they'll likely want to stay at home. The challenge is doing so safely and without becoming isolated when getting out is difficult.

Living at home can be a viable option for your parent. Let's discuss a few strategies, resources, and products to make it work, even if your parent lives alone, has physical challenges, or suffers from mild memory deficits.

Universal Design

One of the first things you can do is to ensure that no structural barriers in the home pose a threat and increase the risk of falling. Many newer homes today, especially in the senior housing industry, use features known as *universal design*.

Definition

Universal design elements fit the needs of everyone at every age—a one-size-fits-all approach. Every room is thus comfortable and safe, and provides convenient access and ease of use for everyone. When done well, universal design is a natural and stylish part of the home—it doesn't scream "handicapped!"

If you want to give your parent a universally designed home, here are features Mom or Dad will appreciate:

- No-step entries into the home, to the backyard, or into the garage
- Wide entries, to accommodate a wheelchair
- Light switches and electrical outlets that are easy to reach
- A main-floor bathroom
- Lever-style door handles and faucets that are painless to grip
- Bathrooms with grab bars, raised toilets, and walk-in tubs or showers

- Raised front-loading laundry machines

- Pull-out shelving in the kitchen and storage areas

- Adjustable cupboards that can be lowered for easy reach

- Lazy Susan turntables

- Counters with open space underneath so that Mom or Dad can sit while preparing food

- Covered entries, to protect against inclement weather

- Good lighting throughout the home

- Single-floor living, when possible

- An electrical stair climb for multiple stories

If upgrading and remodeling is too expensive, given your parent's current income, consider a reverse mortgage to finance the costs. A reverse mortgage is a loan against the home for homeowners age 62 or older that requires no repayment for as long as your parent lives there. It's insured by the Federal Housing Administration.

Tip

AARP has been in the forefront promoting universal design for older homeowners for over a decade. Go to www.aarp.org and enter "universal design" on the search bar to access the Home Fit Guide, a Safety Checklist, tips on hiring contractors, and much more.

AARP also offers a wealth of information and a video on reverse mortgages. On its home page, select Money and then enter the key words "reverse mortgage" in the search bar.

High-Tech Services and Devices

Speaking of universal, just about every older person living alone has one underlying fear—a fall resulting in a broken hip or caused by a stroke that renders the person helpless. A personal emergency response system (PERS) can lay your and your parent's fears to rest. A PERS is a small pendant worn around the neck or wrist. If a person falls or feels sick and needs help, he or she pushes a button on the device that transmits a call to a 24/7 monitoring service. An operator speaks to the user through a base unit and can dispatch emergency help if needed. A new PERS by Phillips Lifeline (www. lifelinesys.com) has an advanced feature with an embedded sensor that detects the trajectory of a fall and automatically activates the call. So if the user has a stroke or becomes unconscious from a fall, emergency help can be summoned without pushing the button. Expect more companies to offer this type of feature.

Home health-care agencies, hospitals, and a wide range of companies like Phillips offer PERS devices, also known as Medical Alerts. The price for the service ranges from $30 to $55 per month.

Electronic Medication Dispensers

One out of ten hospital readmissions of the elderly is due to a medication error. If your parent takes multiple medications and has no one to remind him or her or to help sort through daily prescriptions, this product can keep Mom or Dad out of the hospital. Typically, a caregiver fills the electronic dispenser with an average of one month's supply of medications. A voice-activated reminder or alarm alerts the user that it's time to take his or her pills and dispenses the accurate amount.

You can find these devices by entering "electronic medication dispensers" for an online search, or ask your local pharmacy whether it sells them. Lifeline Systems (another Philips product) sells a dispenser that notifies caregivers by phone message or text if a family member has not taken the pills when dispensed. You can view this product at www.lifelinesys.com or call 1-800-543-3546.

Sensors for Stove Safety

Kitchen fires occur every eight minutes in North America, and seniors are the most likely group to cause them. Fires usually result from distracted users who forget that they have a pan heating up on the stove. The Safe-T-element is an electronically controlled solid-cover plate installed on top of your existing stovetop burner. A control unit inside the stove controls the temperature of the plate, allowing it to reach a maximum of 662°F and preventing grease, food, or clothing from igniting. These devices are being installed in senior housing units and university dorms nationwide. For example, you can purchase a four-burner unit for $180 and arrange for an installer to hook it up for about $60 by calling Pioneering Tech at 1-800-433-6026. To view a brochure, go to www.pioneeringtech.com.

Another device that serves the same purpose is a motion detector that continuously monitors activity in the kitchen. If no movement is detected, the unit's internal timer is activated. When the preprogrammed time is up, the burners on an electric stove automatically turn off. You can find it at the Alzheimer's Store, www.alzstore.com, or call 1-800-752-3238.

Activities of Daily Living Remote Monitors

A growing number of companies offer remote monitoring systems that strategically place wireless sensors throughout the home to pick up motion. This determines, for example, whether a person has taken medicine, gotten out of bed, gone to the bathroom, or left a door open. The system can be programmed to alert a family member or caregiver by phone or text message if there is a change in routine or health status. The caregiver can also access a secure web page to see how the loved one is doing on all measures over a period of time. An online search is your best bet for finding these up-and-coming businesses—enter key words "remote health monitoring."

Telehealth Devices

Every day, my 91-year-old father who lives alone lets his nurse at the Veterans Administration know how he's feeling by answering a series of questions on a touchpad screen. He steps on an electronic scale, which sends his weight to the nurse. Another device reads his blood pressure. If he had diabetes, he could take his blood glucose readings and even have an EKG reading sent to her. If the nurse sees a problem, she calls my dad and me and has him come in for a full exam.

Thousands of older people who live alone are benefiting from telehealth devices like this. (In my dad's case, the VA provides it.) If your parent has a health condition that should be monitored daily, ask his or her doctor to prescribe this type of service. Call your local home health-care agencies to determine whether they or another health-care provider offers it.

High-Touch Human Services

On the high-touch side, a number of services can assist in your parent's daily life. Social services, transportation, home-delivered meals, and health-care services can be provided by your local Area Agency on Aging, given certain income limits.

Call Eldercare Locator at 1-800-677-1116 to find an agency nearest your parent. If your parent is enrolled as a beneficiary of the Veterans Administration, he or she might qualify for similar services. Go to www.va.gov or call 1-800-827-1000 for more information.

Nonmedical senior care is another option. Private companies such as Home Instead Senior Care, Comfort Keepers, and Visiting Angels can help with chores, assist with baths, make meals, shop for groceries, remind care receivers to take their medications, perform light housekeeping, and provide companionship. They can also drive your parent to doctor's appointments. You can find them in the phone book under "Home Care" or "Home Health Care," or search online using keywords "nonmedical senior care."

The bottom line is that living at home independently is more viable than ever by combining high-touch with high-tech services and making a few modifications to home sweet home.

Independent Living Communities

Independent living is what the name implies—residents live on their own, whether in a campus setting, in an apartment building (sometimes referred to as congregate housing), or as part of a continuing care retirement community (CCRC). These types of housing developments focus on providing residents an active, social lifestyle without the hassle of owning a home. Recreational activities, meals served in a restaurantlike setting, transportation, and housekeeping services are core offerings of most senior living communities. Be aware that residents usually pay for these services beyond their monthly rent or mortgage.

A range of options exist in terms of rentals or ownership. Some offer typical apartment rentals with leases. Others require purchasing the property and include a homeowner's fee to cover maintenance costs. Nonprofit groups, religious communities, and for-profit companies operate independent living communities. Most are not regulated by any government agency, and the housing owner does not provide health-care or custodial services.

The U.S. Department of Housing and Urban Development (HUD) has built apartment buildings for seniors in communities throughout the country. Known as Section 202 housing, these options are for people 62 years and older. Beyond providing affordable apartments, the buildings offer supportive services such as meals in a dining room. Community social service agencies often offer services on site and have a referral relationship with the agency that runs the facility. Call Eldercare Locator at 1-800-677-1116 to find the Section 202 Housing nearest your parent. Be aware that there usually is a long waiting list.

Now let's go back to those CCRCs. If your parent can afford the high entry fee ($100,000 to $300,000) and the monthly outlay, life-care communities offer an entire continuum of care, from independent living to skilled nursing care all on one campus. They offer a wide range of activities: golf, swimming, exercise equipment, physical therapy, banking services, educational courses, and transportation.

If residents of these communities become ill, they're able to receive most of their health care on site; when they recover, they can go back to their original residence. For people who enjoy living in a community of peers and want the security of a one-stop approach to long-term care in a campus setting, a CCRC is a perfect match.

So what should you and your parent be looking for? First, research the CCRC's financial solvency. Because your parent will be investing most of his or her life savings in the CCRC, you'll want to make sure that the company has a solid past and promising future. In many states, the Department of Insurance regulates and licenses CCRCs. The community must give prospective residents a "disclosure statement" containing information about the financial status and operation of the facility. Ask for it along with a copy of the latest inspection report.

CCRCs basically offer three types of agreements:

- **Type A extensive agreement.** Beyond housing, residential services, and amenities, this includes unlimited health-related and long-term nursing care for little or no substantial increase in your parent's usual monthly payments.

- **Type B modified agreement.** Beyond housing, residential services, and amenities, a specified amount of long-term nursing home care is included. Once your parent has used the limit, he or she is responsible for paying the bill in full. Remember that Medicare does not cover nursing home care.

- **Type C fee-for-service agreement.** Beyond housing, residential services, and amenities, no health-care or nursing home coverage is included. Your parent is required to pay the bill out of pocket at fee-for-service rates.

Your parent will be asked to sign a detailed contract. It's smart to have both a lawyer and a financial consultant read it over, too. But before they get that far, your parent should spend significant time at the CCRC by going there for lunch and dinner, attending events, and staying overnight for a few days to really get a feel for the community. Here are some questions to ask:

- Who decides what level of care I'll need if I become ill?

- What kind of refund policy do you offer and under what circumstances?

- Are there health insurance requirements? (For example, will the CCRC purchase long-term care insurance on my behalf? If so, with whom?)

- What is the payment schedule? Will I own or rent my residence?

- What are your licensing requirements by the state? Are there any inspection reports, and may I see them?

You can likely get a directory of all the CCRCs in the state by contacting your state's Insurance Department. Most directories provide a brief description of each facility, the entrance fee, and monthly fees, along with contact information. Check out your state's home page to see whether the Department of Insurance provides a directory online.

Be sure to ask whether the CCRC is accredited by the Commission on Accreditation of Rehabilitation Facilities, or CARF (www.carf.org). Accreditation is voluntary, and not all CCRCs opt to go through the process, but it's a good marker of quality. You can view a list of accredited CCRCs in the country by going to CARF's website. It also offers helpful consumer tools to use when looking for a CCRC.

Assisted Living

This type of housing provides residents with services that assist them with the tasks of daily living, such as providing meals, housekeeping, laundry, and medication reminders. The facility might also assist with grooming, bathing, managing bills, and providing transportation. You'll often hear these services referred to as ADLs, for activities of daily living.

Sometimes you'll run into other terms that refer to assisted living, such as residential care, custodial care, or personal-care homes. Assisted living makes sense for your parent if he or she needs assistance in performing the tasks of daily living. Family members also seek this type of living arrangement when they feel it's no longer safe for Mom or Dad to live alone.

Not all assisted living facilities take people with Alzheimer's disease or other forms of dementia. If they do, they offer specialized floors with professional and additional staff to accommodate their needs. If you are looking at such a facility, make sure it is qualified to care for someone with dementia by asking for certification papers it has received from the state regulating agency. Also ask the facility to describe the training its staff has received to care for people with dementia.

Don't assume that your parent is receiving a great deal of one-on-one attention at the facility. It might have a person or two on site 24/7, but it isn't providing direct care to every single resident. Be sure to ask what services are included in the monthly rate. Many facilities have a long list of fees for services you might think are included under the category of assisted living.

Unlike with nursing homes, regulations governing assisted living facilities are uneven and determined by each state. Be sure to ask every facility you visit whether it has a state license, and if so, ask for a copy of any reports the agency issues on the facility. You can also go on that state agency's website to see whether it provides reports online.

Some assisted living facilities have voluntarily gone through an accreditation process and are listed at the website of the Rehabilitation Accreditation Commission, at www.carf.org. Consider it a good sign if the facility has achieved this distinction. But also be aware that other good facilities might not have gone through the arduous process.

Skilled Nursing Facilities

Also known as nursing homes, these facilities provide 24-hour nursing care because residents demand much higher levels of care than those residing in assisted living. For example, more than half of all residents in U.S. nursing homes have dementia and/or lack bowel and bladder control; 80 percent and more have great difficulty bathing, walking, eating, and transferring; and nearly half of the residents are 85 years of age and older.

Nursing homes offer skilled nursing care, rehabilitation, medical services, and protective supervision, as well as assistance with the ADLs. People with long-term mental or physical conditions that require a 24-hour protective environment offering medical and health-care services need nursing home care.

Don't assume that your parents will never need this level of care or that somehow you'll keep them out of a nursing home. Today many nursing homes offer rehabilitative care following a hip fracture, stroke, or heart attack. Patients are being discharged earlier from hospitals than they have in the past and often require a posthospitalization stay at a nursing home to recuperate. So it's in everyone's best interest—while your parent is well—to visit and research local nursing homes.

You and your parents should decide *now* where they want to receive this level of care. You'll make a much smarter decision than waiting for a social worker to show up at your mom or dad's bedside cheerfully announcing, "Good news, you'll be leaving tomorrow."

The following story concerns finding the right level of care for my mother.

When my mother fell and broke her leg while she was still recovering from a broken shoulder, I was forced to find her a skilled nursing facility with a rehab center because the hospital would not admit her. She required two people to assist her whenever she needed to go to the bathroom and get in and out of a chair or bed. We both felt she'd be safer at a rehab center, and so did her doctor. I did all the research like I'm advising you to do, and the reports turned out just fine. In fact, they were very good. But my mom also limited my search and told me not to consider the one other facility near her.

It turned out that my mother's opinion was based on information and a visit she had made five years earlier. It was now under new management and turned out to be far superior than the facility we chose. After just two nights witnessing poor levels of care, I removed my mother from the skilled nursing facility. After more research and a visit to the center she had previously rejected, my mother was pleasantly surprised and decided to go there after all. The care was excellent, and she thrived the six weeks she resided there.

Lessons learned? My mother and I both wished we had visited all the skilled nursing centers in her community while she was well. Though we had a very good home health agency in the wings in case she needed it, we hadn't considered nursing home care. Making that decision during a crisis made us both feel pressured, and we'd relied on outdated and faulty information that had limited her choices.

Second, always, always spend time with your loved one late at night and on weekends at a skilled nursing facility—that's when you'll observe its true levels of care and staff performance. This lesson I did follow and am sure glad I did.

Research Nursing Homes

Your first step in researching nursing homes should be to go online. If you don't have access to the internet, it's worth a trip to your local library to do so, or ask a family member or friend to look up the information for you.

The Centers for Medicare and Medicaid (CMS) requires annual inspections of all nursing homes and posts its five-star ratings on these homes at www.medicare.gov. On the home page, choose Quality Care Finder. You are able to search and compare nursing homes by zip code, county, and state. Contact information, type of ownership (for example, for-profit, nonprofit, or public), number of beds, and whether the facility accepts Medicare and/or Medicaid are also given. The five-star ratings are issued for three categories: health inspection results, nursing home staffing ratios, and quality measures.

You can review the individual results for each of these categories by clicking the name of the nursing home. You can see how the nursing home fares against state and national averages among specific measures and see whether a deficiency has placed residents in danger of harm, on a four-point scale from "least" to "actual."

Look for homes that are no less than average on all measures, when compared to facilities in the state or nation. Measures that should be of special interest to you are staffing levels, use of physical restraints, pressure sores, catheter use and urinary tract infections, weight loss, medication errors, and infection control. Facilities that have a pattern of placing residents at risk for "most" or "actual" harm on quality of care measures are absolute red flags.

After you narrow your search from reviewing Medicare's reports, go to your state's website of the agency that licenses nursing homes. Some states post actual survey reports and more detailed information than the Medicare.gov site, so it's worth a look.

All these steps provide great information—on paper—to assess the quality of care at the nursing home. But there's nothing like making your own site visit. Here's where instincts and an observant eye make a powerful combination. Even better, bring a friend or family member with you.

Tip

Every nursing home is assigned an "ombudsman," usually employed by an Area Agency on Aging or an objective, third-party organization contracted by the agency. An ombudsman helps solve issues, concerns, and problems among residents, their families, and the staff of the long-term care facility. Ask the nursing home for the contact information of the ombudsman, or call 1-800-677-1116 (Eldercare Locator) for the local Area Agency on Aging.

Ask the ombudsman whether there has been any recent complaint activity about the facility and whether it has an ongoing record of consistent deficiencies.

Medicare.gov also provides a Nursing Home Visit Checklist that you can print and take with you. To get you started, here's my own checklist of what to look for:

- ❏ Does it feel like home? Do you feel good about the facility as soon as you walk in?

- ❏ Is the staff interacting in a friendly manner with each other and the residents?

- ❏ Is the facility free of odors? Is it clean? Well lit?

- ❏ Is the temperature comfortable? Stop by a few rooms to see. Many older folks like their rooms warm—is it too cold?

- ❏ Are residents well groomed? Are they dressed appropriately for the time of day? Do they look sedated?

- ❏ Where are the residents? In halls? In group activity rooms? In their rooms appearing isolated?

- ❏ Is there a wandering alert system?

- ❏ Is there an activity calendar? Are there pictures on the bulletin boards showing recent activities? Are the activities interesting and varied?

- ❏ Are there active volunteers helping out?

- ❏ Are lavatories clean? How do they smell?

- ❏ Are food trays left sitting out? Do you see a lot of leftover food on the trays?

❏ Usually above each room in the hallway is a light alerting staff that a resident has pushed a call button for help. How many are lit up, and for how long do they stay lit?

❏ View the menus. Are the meals appetizing? What are the qualifications of whomever oversees the menus? Taste the food.

❏ Are there any safety hazards (for example, cluttered halls or a lack of ramps, rails, or grab bars to prevent falls)?

❏ Does the equipment look up-to-date and in good condition?

❏ Is the outdoor area secure so that no one can wander off into an unsafe area? Is it well landscaped?

❏ Go to the dining room. Are residents enjoying themselves? Is it pleasant? Is staff interacting with the residents?

❏ Are bed linens and towels cleaned daily? Ask what the laundry department does to prevent pressure sores.

❏ Are soiled linens piled up in the hallways or in residents' rooms?

❏ Are showers clean? Look for safety devices to prevent falls.

❏ Is there fresh water on nightstands easily accessible for residents?

❏ How comfortable and homey are the rooms? Do residents personalize them with their own pictures, artifacts, and small furniture?

Consider the Costs

One devastating myth is the belief that Medicare covers nursing home care. With the annual price tag hovering at $80,000 a year, it's a myth that every family wishes were true. But it's not. Medicare *might* cover up to 100 days after an immediate hospitalization that required three nights at a hospital. But that's it. Most people entering nursing homes begin paying with their own funds, but it doesn't take long for them to "spend down" all of their wealth. Many must turn to the state for financial assistance through Medicaid. This explains why more than 60 percent of residents in nursing homes rely on Medicaid as their primary source of payment.

If your parents have a long-term care policy, it will surely help, but it rarely covers the full cost of care. Ask the admissions staff to give you a complete list of all its charges and an explanation of the refund policies if it requires a deposit in advance. Read its contract carefully, especially language that speaks to the rules on discharge and how long it will hold a room for your parent if he or she becomes hospitalized. Don't accept any language that exempts the facility from being held responsible for injuries, falls, or missing belongings.

Alternative Living Arrangements

Besides the living options we've already reviewed, there are a growing number of creative and evolving senior living possibilities that your parents might want to entertain.

Group Homes

This living option caters to people who want a watchful eye looking out for them, like a small homelike setting; don't want to live alone; and might need some daily assistance. They are known by a variety of names: adult family homes, personal-care homes, adult foster homes, group homes, or board-and-care homes. Even though some assisted living facilities are also called "personal-care homes," group homes are much smaller (3 to 10 people) and seldom are regulated or licensed in many states. Frequently, they have fewer than the number of rooms that require any type of oversight in their particular state.

Typically, group homes charge a monthly rate that includes room and board, three meals per day, housekeeping, and laundry services. Some group homes also provide their residents activities and transportation. There's a great deal of variance in what a group home offers and the level of the owner's experience in caring for an older population. If your mom or dad favors this kind of setting, you really need to research the background of the owner and how well residents fare at the group home. You won't have federal or state survey reports to guide you, but you could call local senior centers and ask the director and participants whether they've heard anything about the home. Also ask the Area Agency on Aging's ombudsman, local church, synagogue, and family service agencies. It would also be wise to check with the Better Business Bureau.

Interview the owner and ask for references, along with verification of any training he or she has received. If the owner employs staff to assist, ask what type of background checks he or she performs before hiring anyone. Read the contract carefully and be specific in what is covered. Request to have lunch or dinner with the residents so you can assess how people get along and whether this is the best fit for your mom or dad.

<table>
<tr><td>Alert</td><td>If your parent lives in a group home, make weekly visits to see how things are going. If you live a long distance away, find a local friend of your parent, a neighbor, or a church volunteer. You might even want to hire someone to look in on your mom or dad, to assure you that his or her care is both good and safe.</td></tr>
</table>

ECHO Housing

These backyard cottages work well if you have the land and your parents want to live on their own yet near you. Known as an Elder Cottage Housing Opportunity (ECHO), this is a modular home that can be temporarily placed on your property. They are much smaller (for example, 500 to 800 square feet) than a typical modular home and feature a handicapped-accessible kitchen, bathroom, and living room. They come in a variety of designs that can match the architecture of your home and neighborhood. Make sure you find out what local zoning laws apply before you embark on this project. The average cost ranges from $25,000 to $50,000. Of course, cost can be greater for higher-end elder cottages. To find a backyard cottage, search online using keywords "elder cottage housing" or "ECHO housing." Local companies that sell modular homes are also a good source.

Natural Occurring Retirement Communities (NORC)

These residential areas of single-family homes or apartment complexes were never intended to become senior housing communities. But as people raised their families, got older, and stayed, they "aged in place," and now the community consists mostly of older people—at least 50 percent.

Community planners have seized upon these naturally evolved elder communities and have organized supportive services such as clinics, transportation, meals, social services, recreational activities, and nonmedical senior care so that the residents, many of whom need assistance, can remain there.

Your parent might be living in such a community or apartment building and not even realize it. Call your local Area Agency on Aging to see whether services are available where your parent resides or whether a community service organization would consider organizing one if your parent's building or neighborhood qualifies as a NORC.

Moving Made Easy

Leaving a family homestead is never an easy venture, at any age. But it is especially difficult leaving behind long-held memories that both you and your parent likely share. Realtors and professional organizers can make the move less daunting because they'll organize a sale of furniture, figure out what to bring to new living quarters, assist with the actual move, and even help design the new living space.

You can find professional organizers by visiting the National Association of Professional Organizers at www.napo.net to find a member near you. Also check with your local real estate agents to see whether they offer the service.

Professional organizers offer the following tips to help older parents during a move: Encourage them to choose five of the most important pieces of furniture that will make them feel at "home" at their new place. Take photos of furniture, paintings, and artifacts that have special meaning; then write down the story behind it on a piece of paper and either place it inside the item or tape it to the back so that future generations know its story. Get your parents into the swing of moving by starting with items in the basement that can be given away or sold. Your parent likely won't be emotionally attached to them, so the process of "letting go and moving on" can begin.

Essential Takeaways

- Most older people want to remain in their homes. With assistive devices, telehealth technology, and nonmedical senior care, they can live safely at home.

- Skilled nursing facilities might also provide temporary rehabilitation care due to an injury, a stroke, a heart attack, or surgery following hospitalization. It's not always a permanent placement.

- Assisted living facilities and group homes offer good alternatives for people who need help with the activities of daily living, but many are unregulated and require steadfast monitoring on your part to ensure that your parent is receiving quality care.

chapter 8

Common Legal Matters and How to Work Through Them

The conversation you know you need to have with your parents

Lawyers who specialize in the care of the elderly

The power of attorney and durable health-care power of attorney lawyers

Writing wills, trusts, and letters of instruction

Understanding the laws of guardianship

What "do not resuscitate" means

Many surveys show that American families avoid getting their affairs in order. A "Planning for Your Heirs" poll by the web's leading collector of financial rate material, Bankrate, found that three quarters of respondents believe that everyone should have a will, but more than half of them (57 percent) didn't follow their own advice.

The good news is that the likelihood of having a will increases with age (50-plus); however, nearly 40 percent of the people in that age bracket don't have one, either. Why? They plan to just "let [the] family figure it out." And that response, warns many a financial planner, spells disaster.

So let's prevent a disaster for your family by laying out a plan and initiating it with a much needed conversation.

Having *That* Conversation with Your Parents

All too often, that talk you and your parents have been meaning to have comes in the midst of a health crisis. But when emotions are running high and your parents are fighting for their health, they could not have picked a worse time to make legal decisions. Whether it's quickly putting together a will, figuring out who should make health-care decisions, or deciding how to protect their assets, none of these decisions will be given the attention or research they require.

Some parents hesitate to talk about a will and other legal documents because it's a sign that their role in the family is changing and diminishing, or they interpret the discussion as a signal that their health is declining and they are becoming more dependent. Or maybe they feel that it's bad manners to talk about personal finances—on their part and yours.

Even if your parents have taken the steps to write a will, it's helpful to know what they have planned. If they haven't taken those steps, then broaching the topic, so they can protect their assets and keep peace in the family, is worthwhile.

Here are some tips to help you begin the conversation and what to discuss once you've begun:

- Open the conversation by explaining to your parents that you want to know what *they* want. Try something like, "Mom and Dad, I really want to carry out your wishes, but I need to better understand them. Some people use a will to pass down property, some want to draw down money to help meet costly health-care bills, and others use estate planning to avoid high taxes and lengthy *probate*. What do you want? Is there any way I can be helpful?"

- Let your parents know that planning tools like a will, advance directive, power of attorney, and durable health-care power of attorney will keep *them* in control, not the government or court-appointed strangers through lengthy court proceedings. Nor is this about you taking over. So be sure to stay focused on your parents' concerns, not what you want from them or for them.

- One way of subtly approaching the issue is to share your experience of setting up a will or doing your own estate planning. Perhaps you've learned strategies from your lawyer to better protect your assets, or you've read an article that you can share. Try something like, "Mom, I just filled out a durable health-care power of attorney for my husband, Ben. It was really easy—here's how it works …." Or you could share an actual story of someone's lack of a will that caused a great deal of family friction and lost family wealth to taxes, lawyers, and probate.

- Throughout the conversation, acknowledge that you realize this is *their* money—not yours. Emphasize that they should use their assets to enjoy a good quality of life and to care for each other, in case either of them becomes sick. If they openly discuss their intent to leave you and your siblings an inheritance, certainly be appreciative, but again, reinforce that their careful savings has led to their ability to care for themselves, and that, too, is a gift. It's unfortunate to see older people not spend their money to properly care for themselves because they want to leave it all to their children.

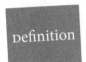

Definition

Probate is a court in which creditors of the person who has died are paid and in which the estate is divided among the heirs after death. This is the court that also administers any estates without wills.

If your parents are uncomfortable talking about this with you, share names of elder law attorneys and financial estate planners that can assist them. Just remember that when all is said and done, an inheritance is a *gift*, not a right.

Elder Law Attorneys

During the last decade, a cadre of new lawyers known as elder law attorneys have burst onto the scene. In the early days, much of their work centered on estate planning for people who wanted to protect their assets against exorbitant nursing home costs.

As the aging population exploded, health care needs expanded, life spans increased, and health-care laws became more complex by the day, the role of and demand for elder care lawyers has grown exponentially. Family dynamics brought on by divorce, remarriage, and blended families has also placed these lawyers smack dab in the middle of family disputes as they help families mediate a wide range of elder care issues.

Most elder law attorneys have undergone special training to understand the needs of the elderly and their families, beyond all the technical and legal expertise they have gained in elder law. Because of their interest in serving a geriatric population, they've learned how to relate to an older clientele, their spouses, and their families. These attorneys can assist with a wide range of legal matters, such as administering and managing trusts; writing wills; fighting for pension, retirement, and disability benefits; drafting power of attorney, durable health-care power of attorney, conservatorships, and guardianship papers; and appealing insurance denials, including Medicare and Medicaid rulings.

And if your parent has been scammed, elder law attorneys can help recover losses or regain credit when an identity thief absconds with their good credit or Social Security number.

MISC.

Finding an Elder Law Attorney

The National Academy of Elder Law Attorneys lists, by location, elder law lawyers and cites which of those are certified in elder law at www.naela. org. The National Elder Law Foundation offers the only national certification of Certified Elder Law Attorneys (CELA) that's approved by the American Bar Association. Visit its site at www.nelf.org to find certified lawyers in your state.

Your state and local bar association, listed in the Yellow Pages of your phone book, is another source for elder law lawyers. You can ask for referrals from geriatric care managers, hospital social workers, and your local senior center.

An internet search with key words "elder law lawyer or attorney" should yield a good number of responses for lawyers in your area.

When you've narrowed your search, you'll want to ask the lawyer a number of questions:

- How long have you been practicing elder law?

- Have you received any special training in elder law?

- Do you have a CELA (Certified Elder Law Attorney) designation? Do you belong to any professional organizations?

- What percentage of your practice is dedicated to elder law?

- What are your specialties in elder law (for example, Medicaid and Medicare denials, estate planning, disability and insurance claim appeals, elder abuse and recovery)?

- Is there a charge for a consultation?

When you meet with the lawyer, be sure to prepare and organize all your parent's materials according to what you want the lawyer to address, and then ask:

- How do you propose to address my parent's case or needs?

- Are there any other courses of action? What are the pros and cons of each?

- How much time do you think it will take to resolve and address this matter?

- Can you project the success rate, based on cases similar to my parent's? Or how will my parent's needs be met with the work you propose?

- Will you be handling my parent's work, or will another attorney— and if so, what is his or her experience with such issues?

Most elder law attorneys do not work on a contingency basis and charge for the initial meeting, so be sure to ask what the fee is before meeting. If you will be placing the lawyer on retainer, carefully read over the retainer agreement before signing. And don't be shy about asking for references of clients who use his or her services.

General Power of Attorney

The irony of this term is that it implies that you need an attorney. But in actuality, you don't—the term *attorney* actually means "agent." A general power of attorney document provides a vehicle for one person (the principal) to authorize another person (the agent) to handle his or her business and personal matters. But depending on how complex those transactions are, you might be smart to use a lawyer, after all.

Powers of attorney, for example, can pay bills, handle checking and savings accounts, make decisions on renovating property, or whatever else the principal wants them to do. The principal can spell out the range of decision-making responsibilities the agent has and on what matters in the document. The power given to an agent can be revoked at any time, whereas the principal remains competent.

There are basically four types of power of attorney:

- General durable power of attorney remains in effect for the duration of the principal's life. When the principal dies, it is no longer in effect. (This is when the executor of a will takes over.) It stays in effect, even if the principal becomes incompetent from a stroke, for example. In this event, it saves the family from seeking court action to handle the principal's affairs. As long as the principal is competent, either he or she can make a decision and manage the business and personal matters, or he or she can ask the power of attorney to do so.

- Nondurable power of attorney remains in effect during a specified period of time. It terminates if the principal becomes incapacitated.

- Springing power of attorney "springs" into action at a specific start date or specification of an event or condition. In this instance, the principal can specify that the agent has power when he or she *is* incapacitated.

- Limited power of attorney is in effect for only the duration of time needed to carry out specific purposes, with given start and end dates cited in the document.

The power of attorney must follow the laws of the state where the agent will carry out his or her duties. Your parent can identify co-agents who must act in agreement in fulfilling his or her duties and co-sign all transactions.

Your parent has several options on what kind of power of attorney vehicle meets his or her needs. In any event, it's a resource your parent and you should use.

Durable Health-Care Power of Attorney

Durable health-care power of attorney is broader than a living will or advance directive (see Chapter 12). It empowers an "agent," appointed by the individual signing the document, to make health-care decisions on the person's behalf in case he or she becomes incompetent. This agent can make decisions on admissions to and discharges from health-care facilities, gain access to medical records, determine whether to authorize an organ donation, authorize whether to move the patient, make arrangements for home health care, and accept or refuse treatment that affects the physical and mental health of the patient. These medical decisions come into play at all levels of health care—not just when death is imminent.

You don't have to be a lawyer to be designated as durable health-care power of attorney. The word *attorney* simply means "designated agent." The power of attorney takes effect only when an individual is determined to be legally incompetent. For example, your dad might not be able to communicate following a stroke or might be too confused following surgery to make decisions. In that case, you'll be the one to decide whether it's safe for him to go home or what home health-care agency to hire to help him with his recovery. However, as soon as he has recovered and is competent, your father resumes the power to make his own health-care decisions. Your parent must sign the durable health-care power of attorney when he or she is competent and in front of a witness.

The following is a story about how durable health-care power of attorney prevented a crisis for my father and our family.

In his late 80s, my sharp-as-a-tack father had intestinal surgery and had a severe reaction to the anesthesia. Within 12 hours, he became delusional: he saw trucks speeding down the hospital halls, imagined snow in his hospital room, and accused the hospital of taking over his home. He was appalled at the nurses for rudely refusing to knock on the door of *his* home. He was also upset that I allowed the hospital to take over his property. For three days, my dad needed 'round-the-clock "Safety Sitters" at night because he was pulling out IVs and was a danger to himself. I stayed by his side 12 hours a day, and it was the most exhausting three days of my life.

There's a term for what he went through—postoperative cognitive dysfunction (POCD). Anesthesia can cause this disorder in advanced-aged elderly. The neuropsychologist who examined my father reported seeing people suffer from POCD from three months to a year. In extreme cases, the condition can't be reversed. The nurses on the surgical floor were so familiar with POCD that they were the ones who decided to use nurse aides as "Safety Sitters." One group told me the hospital puts boxing gloves on older patients with POCD so they don't harm themselves.

Because I had durable health-care power of attorney, I was able to arrange the care my father needed for the next two weeks while he regained his mind and his health. My sister and I took shifts staying with him until he was able to be on his own. As his mind wrestled back from the effects of POCD, he recalled what it was like to "go nuts" and begged me to never let that happen again.

I met with the anesthesiologist on duty and asked whether my father could be given another type of anesthesia if he ever needed surgery in the future. Today my dad wears a bracelet indicating that he's allergic to Etomidate and that, when he did need surgery four weeks later due to a postoperative adhesion, he had no such reaction to the anesthesia (Propofol).

Having durable health-care power of attorney prevented a serious problem for my father and our family. What would have happened had he not recovered, or if he needed skilled nursing care in the interim? He was in no condition to make decisions for himself—at that point, he could not sign over any such powers because he was then diagnosed as incompetent. A living will would not have been helpful because he was not dying.

Filling out this simple form can save your family from a world of complex legal and health-care hardship—just do it. By the way, have *you* filled one out?

Every adult should have both a living will and a durable health-care power of attorney. It's far better to thoughtfully and openly consider these issues while you're well than to do so in the midst of an emergency. Furthermore, once your parent is incapacitated, he or she no longer has the option to sign over a power of attorney or durable health-care power of attorney to a family member or any other designee. It will then be too late.

Wills, Letters of Instruction, and Trusts

Wills signify so much more than money; they represent values, the meaning we attribute to property and relationships, and how we view family. Add to all these deeply held feelings the respect for privacy among the Greatest Generation, and it's no wonder so many people avoid the conversation. But *not* having a will can heap a great deal of stress on your family—or even break it apart.

Wills

We've heard the phrase plenty of times: "I, John Smith, being of sound mind, hereby bequeath …." Then away John goes, bestowing his life possessions to family and friends. A will is simply a legal document that provides instructions on how your parent wants property to be passed on to heirs after he or she dies. Witnesses (who don't benefit from the will) are needed, and the will must be in writing and clearly dated. It must also follow state laws.

People write wills, create trusts, and conduct estate planning for three main reasons:

- They want to pass their assets to their family members rather than hand it over to the courts to decide.

- They want to keep peace in the family by preempting squabbles among family members by identifying who gets what when they die.

- They want their wishes to be followed and want to provide for their spouse and children.

Don't consider a will to be written in stone. Families and circumstances change, and so should wills. Many experts recommend that each parent have his or her own will to avoid the complications of a joint one. This is especially true if your parents have remarried.

Wills usually describe assets, property, and personal possessions and how they are to be distributed after someone dies, according to the owner's wishes. Most often the will passes assets to a surviving spouse and then to children. In a will, your parent needs to identify who will administer his or her estate—meaning pay taxes and outstanding bills, and ensure that the instructions in the will are carried out. The person who does this is known as the executor (if a man) or executrix (if a woman).

If your parent dies without a will, it's known as dying intestate. In this instance, the state determines the rightful heirs and how much they receive. The state and Uncle Sam take a greater chunk of your parent's estate than if he or she had a will. Even probate costs are higher. The courts appoint someone to manage the distribution of your parent's estate for a fee. And it takes longer to process than if your parents had a will. You really don't want to end up here.

Tip	Nolo's legal website (www.nolo.com) offers free legal articles, videos, and explanations to all kinds of legal information and do-it-yourself online forms for wills, advance directives, and power of attorney—or you can order CDs. It also has a lawyer search function. Visit the site or call 1-800-992-6656 to order any of the products.

AARP offers its members a free 45-minute consultation with lawyers in partnership with Allstate. If you decide to retain the lawyer, you'll receive a 20 percent discount on the attorney's usual and customary rates. Go to www.aarplsn.com (AARP Legal Services Network) or call 1-866-330-0753.

For seniors with low incomes, contact Eldercare Locator for legal helplines and seek out Legal Aid Societies in communities, at 1-800-677-1116. Or visit the site at www.eldercare.gov; choose "Search by Topic" and then click "Legal Assistance."

Personal Property Memorandum and Letter of Instruction

In addition to a will, some people may write a memorandum of tangible personal property, also known as a personal property memorandum. This is an informal memorandum that describes your parent's wishes to distribute tangible properties such as jewelry, household furniture, dishes, books, paintings, a baseball card collection, or pets that are not listed in the will for disposition. The memorandum is a convenient tool for your parents to list and distribute personal effects without needing to go back and formally amend the will should they change their minds, circumstances change, or they acquire additional items that they want to pass down to a specific heir.

Alert	If your parent writes a personal property memorandum, some states require that it must be referenced in their most recently dated will to make it valid. Your parents may make subsequent changes to the memorandum and when they do, they should sign and date it. State laws govern whether or not and how the memorandum is considered legally binding. Be sure to ask a lawyer as to what your state requires when drafting such a memorandum.

A personal property memorandum provides an extra ounce of prevention against family disputes over the "small stuff." Advise your parent to identify who gets what heirlooms; many an estate lawyer will tell you that the most bitter family feuds are over seemingly insignificant items, like a small piece of furniture, a set of dishes, or an inexpensive piece of jewelry. It's usually something that a family member feels a strong attachment toward because it brings back fond memories of the loved one; to the family, the artifact is priceless and worth the fight. If your parents have thoughtfully identified something that they want each family member to receive, then it's more likely their children will remain friends and won't argue over who gets the ceramic mug collection.

Your parent would also do well to draft a letter of instruction that doesn't require a lawyer and is not part of the will. It does, however, provide instructions that assist heirs in disposition of the will and other matters following death. Here are some examples of what your parent might list:

- Arrangements to care for a pet(s)
- Funeral and burial instructions—what organizations should receive memorial contributions
- The location of important legal documents
- A list of all insurance policies, stocks, beneficiaries, bank accounts, identification of passwords, and PIN numbers
- Instructions regarding credit cards, mortgages, titles of cars, properties, the location of income tax returns, and a list of debts
- Instructions regarding business files, software, equipment, and the password to the computer and online services
- Personal wishes on how your parent would like to see the heirs spend or invest their inheritance

Most beneficiaries respect the wishes of the decedent when they've clearly expressed who they want to receive what in a personal property memorandum, and they are very grateful for a letter of instruction to guide them through the many estate matters following their death.

Trusts

Plenty of people think that trusts are for the rich and famous. But that really isn't so. Basically three types of trusts exist: testamentary, revocable, and irrevocable living trusts. Let's take a closer look at each.

Testamentary Trusts

A testamentary trust is usually established to hold assets for a specific reason, such as a child's college education. This kind of trust comes into effect after your parent's death, as spelled out in the will. Your parent's assets are transferred to the trustee as if that trustee were the beneficiary. The trustee's job is to hold the property for the actual beneficiary. Two major reasons people set up this type of trust are to escape taxes and to provide a means of holding assets until a beneficiary reaches the age of maturity.

Revocable Living Trusts

Revocable living trusts are constructed during your parent's lifetime. Your father or mother retains full control of the trust unless he or she becomes incapacitated. A secondary trustee is also designated—often a bank or other financial institution. If your parent becomes incapacitated, the secondary trustee takes over and follows the directives your parent has outlined in the trust. This way, your parent maintains control. One major advantage is that any property placed in the trust does not go through probate.

It also means that if your dad is diagnosed with Alzheimer's disease, no one has to go through the rigorous legal steps involved in acquiring guardianship. The trust is completely private, whereas wills are public documents. No one can contest a trust as they can a will. Probate costs also are avoided, and your parent can revoke the trust at any time.

Irrevocable Living Trusts

Now enter the rich and famous. People with extremely large estates use irrevocable living trusts. And as the name implies, these trusts can't be changed or destroyed. The grantor sets the terms of the trust during his or her lifetime; however, the grantor can't change those terms once they are set in motion. This is as close to setting something in stone as you can get. If your parent is in the position of being able to consider this option, he or she will certainly have the resources to hire lawyers to execute the trust.

Tip

Wills, advance directives, power of attorney, letters of instruction, personal property memoranda, and other legal documents are worthless if they are hidden away for safe keeping and no one knows how to access them in an emergency or after death. Someone needs to know where these valuable documents are kept. And in cases of living wills and durable health-care power of attorney, copies should be in the hands of those responsible for executing decisions during a health-care crisis.

Guardianship as the Last Resort

At some point, you may face the heart-wrenching point at which your parent severely lacks the capacity to make decisions on his or her behalf or has become a serious threat to him- or herself or others. If your parent is no longer competent to grant you the powers of attorney, you have a hard road ahead when pursuing guardianship.

Seeking guardianship is something you do as a last resort. It is a public court proceeding that imposes demanding rules and tests to determine your parent's capacity to make decisions. You will need to retain a lawyer to petition the court, and the court will appoint a lawyer to represent your parent. Interviews will be conducted with those involved with your parent's care (for example, the family physician); you might bring expert testimony such as the results of a geriatric assessment, or the court might order such an assessment. Your parent will be informed of the hearing and can attend if he or she wants to.

Every state has its own laws governing guardianship. These laws can be rather complicated and might change, thus the need for a lawyer. You'll also find that most states have different levels of guardianship. Limited guardianship, for example, provides the guardian authority over certain limited conditions. For example, Mom might not be capable of handling any of her finances but is capable of making decisions about who takes care of her at home. In most states, guardians usually report to the court at specified times to update the court on how matters are progressing.

If the court declares your parent incompetent or incapacitated, he or she can no longer vote, sell property, execute finances, determine living arrangements and medical treatments, drive, or enter into any type of contracts. Hopefully, you won't have to go down this path, but if you do, work with a lawyer who specializes in elder law and guardianship. Informal agreements among family members can turn bitter very quickly, leaving you open to a wealth of legal problems and even accusations of elder abuse.

Understanding "Do Not Resuscitate" Orders

DNR orders stand for "do not resuscitate." This means that if an individual stops breathing or his or her heart stops beating, no one is to try to revive him or her. In hospitals, the DNR term is also referred to as a "no code." An individual must have signed an advance directive (living will) or other legal document specifying his or her wish not to be resuscitated and under what circumstances. The directive must meet his or her state's legal requirements. A physician writes a DNR order on a patient's medical record, alerting all health-care staff not to resuscitate the patient.

In some states, a living will or advance directive is not effective in the event of a medical emergency involving ambulance personnel. Emergency medical technicians (EMT) and paramedics are required to perform CPR unless they are given separate orders that state otherwise.

These orders are commonly referred to as "nonhospital do-not-resuscitate orders" and are designed for people who are in such poor health that there is little benefit from CPR. These orders should be sought directly from a physician, and you must be prepared to show the papers at the time of an emergency. Your primary care physician should be a good source to learn of your state's requirements. Some states even offer DNR wristbands that can be worn by individuals who have complied with the legal documentation of removing any legal liability against EMTs who have followed their wishes. If your parent chooses this option, make sure that all your family members are aware of it.

Essential Takeaways

- Not having a will places your family in jeopardy not only of financial hardship and loss, but also of fracturing whatever solid foundation and relationships it currently enjoys.

- Power of attorney and durable health-care power of attorney are not the same, nor are their powers interchangeable. Your parents should have both legal instruments.

- Elder law attorneys specialize in issues facing older people. Those who are certified are designated by the initials CELA and have passed a national exam approved by the American Bar Association.

- You can complete many legal documents yourself, and resources are available on the internet to do so. Public resources also provide legal assistance to older people with modest means.

Part 3

Managing Medical Life

If any component of caregiving can overwhelm you, it is handling your parent's health care. Interpreting symptoms, knowing when to call the doctor or schedule an appointment, keeping track of and understanding test results, navigating the world of specialists and body parts medicine, and managing myriad prescriptions are just some of the "medical life" issues you'll encounter.

The other issues? How to pay for long-term care; deal with Medicare, Medigap, and Medicaid; and traverse the fine-print landscape of insurance issues and appeals. And then there's the likely chance that your parent will warrant an emergency-room visit, enter the hospital, and be discharged to a world of home care and rehabilitation. Most of that will turn your world upside down.

Gain control by learning how to prepare for doctor's appointments, share information among physicians and other health-care providers, find the best hospitals and avoid mistakes while your parent is a patient, and know how to stop an early discharge.

Calling in hospice is one of the hardest yet wisest and most compassionate choices you'll ever make. Find out when and how to select a hospice, and acquire insights from those who've traveled this path on what your loved one wants and needs during end-of-life care.

You and your parent's health are intertwined—being overwhelmed endangers both of you.

chapter 9

Getting Organized Medically

Managing your way through the world of specialists

Getting the most out of doctor visits

Reducing your loved one's risk of medication errors

Going digital to organize your parent's medical affairs

There is so much chronic disease among Americans 65 years and older, that the Centers for Disease Control and Prevention now report it as the leading cause of death among the elderly. If you're caring for an aging parent, then you know all too well the challenges of caring for a loved one struggling with chronic disease. The nonstop stream of doctor visits, hospitalizations, prescriptions, medical tests, and directives from multiple doctors is downright overwhelming. It also increases the likelihood that your parent will be the victim of a medical error. It's time to get control, and you'll learn how in this chapter.

Navigating Body Parts Medicine

One of the great advances of the American health-care system is the breadth and depth of knowledge gained by and from physicians who have specialized in a particular branch of medicine. You have a heart problem; you want the best heart doc in town. Think of how many times you've asked friends whether they know of a physician who's excellent at whatever health issue you're facing. (I'm still searching for an absolutely pain-free dentist.)

Most of us feel better knowing that we're seeing someone who has spent years getting to know all the complexities and latest treatments for the part of the body that demands our attention. But what happens when we reach an age when quite a few body parts require quite a bit of attention? The average person in his or her mid-70s struggles with three chronic conditions and takes five prescriptions that send him or her knocking upon many a specialist's door.

An 85-year-old friend of mine, a retired clinical psychologist, told me during his last six months of life while we sat in a waiting room together for his fourth office visit of the week that he was now seeing a nephrologist for his kidney condition, a urologist for his catheter care, a rheumatologist for his gout, a cardiologist for his congestive heart disease, a wound doctor for a sore that wouldn't heal (who he good naturedly renamed a woundologist), and an internist for "none of the above."

He found it dehumanizing. His wife, who had to juggle the six specialists, found it exhausting. His adult children found it frustrating. Even my friend's internist found it difficult to coordinate all the test results and create a plan of care. None of the specialists practiced within one health-care system, so it was essentially up to him and his wife to brief each specialist on his overall health issues, treatment regimen, and medications.

As we move toward electronic health records and consolidated health-care systems, it might become easier to coordinate each individual's health care. But in the meantime, a great deal of the responsibility falls to caregivers. You'll need to organize your loved one's medical records, make sure each doctor is aware of what the others prescribe, and manage appointments.

Speaking of managing appointments, a study appearing in the *Journal of Evaluation in Clinical Practice,* "Errors in completion of referrals among older urban adults in ambulatory care," caught my attention because it exemplifies the fall-out of what I call "body parts medicine." Half of all patients who were referred to a specialist by their primary care doctor never got there! There's a host of reasons for the specialist disconnect: patients didn't follow through, they lacked transportation, they felt too sick to go, the specialist couldn't see them for a month or more and they gave up, the doctor's office faxed the referral to the wrong office, the specialist's office didn't get the fax, or someone forgot to confirm the appointment with the patient.

Whatever the reason, not receiving the specialized care to treat a condition can cause serious problems for elderly patients that could have been prevented, warns Dr. Michael Weiner, lead author of the study. I had a chance to talk with Dr. Weiner, who is also a professor of medicine at the Indiana School of Medicine. He advises that caregivers and patients always ask the doctor certain questions: "Why are you referring me to this specialist, and what do you want to learn from him or her?" Then ask the doctor, "What's the process in getting an appointment, and who handles the follow-up once I've seen the specialist you referred me to?" Then make the appointment!

If your loved one has been given a referral to see a specialist, here are the steps to take:

- If the doctor's office makes the appointment for your parent, ask if you can remain in the waiting area while it's made so you won't have to wonder whether the office followed through.

- If the doctor gives you the name of a specialist to call, ask for the name of a second specialist, in case the first referral no longer accepts new patients or the wait for an appointment is too long.

- Even if the appointment is months away, take the first available appointment—but also ask to be placed on a waiting list for a cancellation. If the office doesn't have a waiting list, ask what number you should call in the mornings to find out whether a cancellation comes up so you can get your parent in sooner.

- If the specialist cannot see your parent for an extended period of time and your doctor feels your mom or dad should be seen quickly, call the physician's office back. Ask whether they think the wait is acceptable or whether they would please intervene and get the appointment moved up.

Tip

At every appointment with a specialist, be sure to bring a current list of medications and a medical biography of your parent's health conditions, allergies, and other physicians he or she sees. You can access Med Minder, Medical Biography, and My Medical Data forms at my website (www.lindarhodescaregiving.com), and they are also shown in Appendix C.

If you can't make an appointment, be sure to call ahead to cancel so that someone else who wants to be seen quickly may be given the opportunity.

Finding a Captain: The Primary Care Doctor

If your parent belongs to a Medicare Advantage plan or health maintenance organization, he or she will likely be assigned a primary care physician (PCP) who will coordinate care among the doctors within the plan's network. If your parent belongs to Original Medicare, then he or she has the option to see any desired doctor; however, no one is directly in charge of your parent's care. That means your mom or dad should find a PCP, family practice doctor, general practitioner, or internist specializing in geriatrics to oversee his or her health care.

PCPs provide preventive care, perform routine screening exams, inform patients of healthy lifestyle practices, identify and treat common medical conditions, assess the urgency of presenting symptoms, and make referrals to medical specialists. When your mother is feeling ill or complains of troubling symptoms that should be checked out, her PCP should be her first point of contact.

It's important that you and your parent have a candid conversation with the PCP to understand what role he or she is willing to perform in terms of coordinating care. The best-case scenario is a physician who will assume the role as captain, to act as the central point of command among all the health-care providers involved in your parent's care. You'll also want the physician to be an assertive advocate whenever obstacles jeopardize that care.

Here are some questions you and your parent should ask the PCP, to determine his or her coordinative role:

- Will you act as my primary liaison with other health-care providers that you refer me to?

- Will you discuss my test results and other pertinent information with other physicians and health-care providers, to develop a collaborative plan of care?

- Will you review all my test results and other medical information sent to you and tell me what they mean?

- How soon can I expect a report on the results? Who should I call if I haven't received them?

- Will your office make appointments to specialists that you refer me to? If not, will you intercede on my behalf if I run into problems securing a timely appointment?

- What can I do to make it easier for you to coordinate my care?

If you are heavily involved in your parent's health care and accompany your loved one to appointments, ask the physician about the best way to communicate with him or her regarding your parent. For example, is email acceptable, or should you call a specific nurse or leave a message at the office? Introduce yourself to the nurse manager, and give her all your contact information and ask that it be placed in your parent's chart. Before you leave the appointment, make sure your mom or dad has signed a HIPAA privacy consent form that allows the doctor to speak to you regarding your parent's health status.

Preparing for Doctor Appointments

Knowing how to work with and relate to your parent's PCP is right up there with getting along with your boss, your co-workers, and, I dare say, even your spouse. Because the PCP is your parent's link to vital health care, if you don't get along with the physician or know how to work with him or her, the link is broken or, at best, weakened.

So wouldn't it help if you knew what makes the doctor happy?

How to Relate to Your Parent's Doctors

Consumer Reports unlocked the answer in a cover story featuring "What doctors wish their patients knew." I thought it was an interesting take on the doctor-patient relationship, since most surveys and reports focus on what patients think of doctors. *Consumer Reports* National Research Center surveyed 660 PCPs from across the country to gain their perspective. So let's take a look at what the doctors had to say.

Three out of four docs said that developing a long-term relationship with a PCP is the most important thing your parents can do to ensure better medical care. Patients who shop around, seeing different doctors without one consistent physician as a captain, can easily fall through the cracks. Symptoms, medications, medical conditions, and test results are puzzle pieces that won't form a whole picture without a PCP putting them together.

Patients like doctors who are courteous and listen. Doctors want the same from their patients, but they report (in 70 percent of cases) that respect and appreciation have gotten "a little worse" or "much worse" since they started practicing medicine. If you want your doctor to respect you and your parent, you'll need to do the same.

Most physicians find it helpful when patients ask questions rather than remain completely passive. It gives them a better understanding of the patient's concerns and ability to follow treatment plans. The docs also said—80 percent of them—that it's helpful to bring someone along to appointments. They welcome a second set of ears and find it reassuring when someone is taking notes. So if your parents want to go it alone, let them know that the doctor actually *wants* you to tag along.

Paperwork Still Matters

Even though most physician practices are moving toward electronic health records (EHR), 9 out of 10 doctors advise that keeping track of your medical history, results of previous doctor visits, health conditions, a list of current medications and any side effects, test results, and a list of other doctors who treat you is extremely helpful.

Do your research, but be careful of what you find on the internet. Nearly half of the doctors said that "online research helps very little or not at all." A mere 8 percent thought it was "very helpful." So if you are going to use online research, stay with reliable sites, such as www.medlineplus.gov; the Mayo Clinic, at www.mayoclinic.org; or national, nonprofit associations on diseases such as www.alzheimers.org. Listen to your doctor first and use the research to ask better-informed questions. Don't walk in with pages of printed online articles showing the doctor what you think he or she should do.

Doctors appreciate patients who realize that they are under a lot of pressure and time constraints. The number one obstacle they said they face is financial issues posed by red tape (42 percent said "a lot") and the sheer volume of insurance paperwork, along with complicated health plans. To maximize your time with your doctor, make a list of key questions before the appointment that you want to ask, and tell the doctor you've prepared a list—that way, the two of you can use the visit wisely.

Not complying with taking medications or following advice on treatment plans is the chief complaint of doctors regarding their patients. They feel that it significantly affects their ability to provide high-quality care. If your parent has side effects to medications or can't afford them, don't hide this information from your doctor. Or if your loved one finds the treatment regimen too complicated or isn't satisfied with it, let him or her know. Ignoring the doctor's advice will make matters worse for the both of you.

What to Ask the Doctor

Far too often, older people feel that they will appear impolite if they ask their doctor questions, or they worry that their questions will sound foolish. So they clam up. But not asking could lead to medical errors by either the patient or the doctor. Misunderstanding the directions on how to take a prescription or not comprehending the risks of a procedure often leads to a troubled outcome that a simple question could have avoided.

A commercial sponsored by the Agency for Healthcare Research and Quality (AHRQ) features a waiter with a voice in the background saying, "You don't have trouble asking him about side dishes," and then pans out to a doctor holding a prescription bottle. The announcer then asks, "So why can't you ask *him* about side effects?" The goal of the ad campaign is to illustrate how often we ask questions in everyday life but go mum in medical settings.

Part of the agency's public awareness campaign is to offer consumers a list of questions to ask their doctors. You can check them out at its website at www.ahrq.gov/questionsaretheanswer and learn more on how to be an informed patient.

Based on the AHRQ's questions and my own experience, here are some questions you or your parent should ask doctors:

- Bring a list of all medications for every doctor to review and ask: Should I continue to take all these? Are there any side effects I should be concerned about? Do any of these medications interact negatively with another? If a new drug is prescribed, use the same questions, but also ask how to spell the drug and what it is for.

- If blood tests, x-rays, scans, or any other diagnostic procedure are prescribed, ask: What are these tests for? When will you know the results? How will you let me know the results? If I haven't heard from you, who should I call at your office to find out the results? Don't assume that no news is good news or accept, "We'll get back to you if there is a problem." You need to know either way.

- If surgery is recommended, ask: What is this surgery for? Can you explain what's done during the surgery, and could you draw or show a picture of it? Is there an alternative that I can try first? What are the possible complications, given my age and health condition? How long will my recovery be, and what can I expect during it? Can you give me two choices of surgeons to see?

- If your parent has been told he or she has a specific health condition, ask: Do you have reading materials on it? Do you have any video or audiotapes I could review? Are there any written instructions I should follow?

- At the end of every office visit, ask the doctor: Could you please tell me what are the two or three most important things I should remember or do as a result of today's exam?

None of these questions should feel off-putting for your parents, and you can reassure them that the doctors will actually appreciate them asking. An informed patient is more likely to follow doctor's orders—and that makes physicians happy campers.

Managing Medications

One of the most common reasons older people end up in emergency rooms—some estimates are as high as 100,000 people a year—is harmful reactions to medications. Drugs that don't work together, negative side effects, and patients who don't follow prescription directions are the leading causes. With nearly one third of all older Americans taking more than five prescription drugs a day, it's no wonder that over 1 million people a year are harmed by a medication error or what medical experts call an adverse drug event (ADE).

As our bodies age, we process medications differently. More body fat, less lean body mass, less total water in the body, lower metabolism, and reduced kidney and liver cleansing function make for a perfect storm of toxic drug build-up. Add to that the numerous ingredients contained in each drug—multiplied by the number of drugs your parent takes—and a fragile geriatric body finds itself hosting a chemical slugfest. Somebody's going to lose.

Physicians are urged to consult a tool known as the Beers Criteria or the Beers List. It identifies medications noted by an expert panel of geriatricians and pharmacologists to have risks that outweigh benefits of the drug for patients 65 years and older. It also alerts physicians of potentially inappropriate medications for older adults, listed by disease or condition. You can access the Beers List and my highlights from it by going to my website and clicking "Caregiver Tips of the Week."

So how do you keep your parents safe and healthy when it comes to prescription use? Besides the medication questions we just reviewed to ask at every doctor's visit, here are 10 safety tips to keep your parents out of harm's way:

1. Look for pharmacies that use bar codes. This safety feature reduces human error so that pharmacy technicians are less likely to take the wrong drug off the shelf and pharmacists are less likely to give the wrong dose.

2. When you buy a drug, herb, or dietary supplement over the counter, stop by and ask the pharmacist his or her opinion on whether it will interact with any of your current prescription medications. It's

smart to keep a list of these medications with you. Just because you can buy a drug without a prescription doesn't mean it is safe.

3. If you have been taking a generic, a pharmacist can substitute your refill with another generic that's different from the first. If you have been satisfied with the generic drug you have been taking, tell the pharmacist.

4. Two out of three patients walk out of their doctor's office with a prescription in hand. When you read the prescription, ask for the spelling of the drug, what it is for, and the dose. Double-check this with the pharmacist and the label on the medicine bottle. Also, don't be afraid to ask your doctor whether there is another solution to your health problem other than taking a pill, to reduce your risks of an ADE.

5. Talk to your pharmacist. According to the Institute for Safe Medication Practices, half of us are taking medications improperly. So ask your pharmacist for any special directions you should follow. And always check with the pharmacist before you crush medicines or cut them in half, because they might be slow-release drugs that should be taken whole.

6. If you are the type of person who will do better taking a pill once a day versus three or four times a day, ask the pharmacist or your physician if the medication you've been prescribed can be given in a way that will be easier for you.

7. Most pharmacies will enter your health history, allergies, and list of medications into a database. That way, they can cross-check any new medications you are prescribed for possible adverse reactions or drug interactions. It's your job to give them this information and keep it up-to-date.

8. If you're home and discover that the labels or directions are confusing to you, call the pharmacy and ask to speak to the pharmacist to explain it to you. Don't guess at what you should do.

9. Don't wait until a prescription has run out before you get a refill, especially if it is a drug that requires you to stay on schedule. The same goes for calling your doctor's office at the last minute for a

refill that has expired. Because of busy schedules and large volumes of prescriptions being filled, you might end up missing a dose.

10. If you notice on a refill that the pill is a different color or shape from what you had before, or if the dose has changed (for example, 10 mg to 100 mg), ask the pharmacist to explain. It could be a mistake.

Patient safety is everyone's responsibility, and that includes consumers. An excellent website on medication safety is www.consumermedsafety. org, sponsored by the Institute for Safe Medication Practices. You can look up thousands of medications, including over-the-counter drugs, to find out what they do and view warnings and side effects, at www. medlineplus.gov.

Now let's talk about how your parents can dispense their pills. In response to the growing problem of elderly wrestling with managing their medications, the National Institute on Aging funded a study to see whether electronic pillboxes help people keep up with their meds and avoid harmful mistakes. They found that these did help: The number of days that people forgot to take their drugs on time dropped in half, and patients were much better at taking the second or third dose of a medicine instead of taking one for the whole day.

You can find a wide range of electronic pill-dispensing and reminder products on the market. The challenge is to find something that won't overwhelm your parent yet will do the job. Here's a quick recap of the kinds of pill-management products you'll find:

- **Reminders:** These devices come in the form of watches, wristbands, or pendants that the patient wears, or clocks and timers that are programmed to beep when he or she needs to take a medication. Many offer voice recordings with pill-taking instructions.

- **"Talking" pill bottles:** These products have a recording device on the bottle, and the patient pushes a button to listen to a message (for example, how many pills to take and how). The pharmacist might have this type of recording unit, or a family member can record the relevant information. There are also "smart bottle caps" with recordings or digital screens that display pill-taking instructions, or bottle holders that do the same when you place the prescription bottle in it.

■ **Electronic pill dispensers:** Dispensers organize all pills, ranging from a week to a month supply. An alarm beeps when it is time to take a medication and automatically dispenses the pills. These often include voice-recorded instructions, and some can be phone-activated so that far-away caregivers and doctor's offices can monitor whether the medications were taken.

An excellent assistive technology information source for these products is AbleData, at www.abledata.com or 1-800-227-0216.

Getting Health-Care Providers on the Same Page

Given that your parents might see a good number of physicians during the course of your caregiving, it will be helpful to prepare a portfolio of information that contains their medical biography, medication list, and emergency contact information. It's also helpful to prepare folders that contain test results and other medical data pertinent to each specialist.

But that's about to change. With the passage of the Affordable Health Care Act, we've entered the era of electronic health records (EHR), also known as electronic medical records (EMR). Physicians, hospitals, and other health-care providers are moving toward using electronic record keeping and sharing of patient medical data. The goal is to improve communication among health-care providers, ensure better coordination and quality of care, and reduce medical errors. Electronic prescribing is also done at doctors' offices, making it easier to avoid mistakenly reading handwritten prescriptions.

A personal health record (PHR) is an electronic, web-based information record of health data that you collect about your health. You control who might have access to it. When you set one up, you receive a unique user identification and can create your own password at a secure, web-based site. So if you'd like to keep all your parent's medical data in one place and share it with doctors and other family members, developing a PHR will be a welcome addition to your caregiving tools. You can list prescriptions, health conditions, and allergies; keep track of doctor's appointments; track email exchanges with family members; collect articles on medical information; and even download Medicare claims data to your PHR. In a medical emergency, you can give emergency medical technicians or hospital staff access to your PHR. If you have a smart phone, you can simply enter data right from a doctor's office or call it up to share with whomever needs to see it.

PHRs are offered by health-care providers, health plans, nonprofit groups, government agencies, and private companies that either offer it for free or charge for the service. For example, the VA Administration offers a PHR for VA patients through MyHealtheVet, and Medicare provides a Blue Button feature through which you can download your Original Medicare claims onto your PHR. MyMedicare.gov allows you to organize your medications, Medicare-certified providers, Medicare Summary Notices, and other health-care information.

The Mayo Clinic offers a free PHR called Mayo Clinic Health Manager; you do not have to be a patient at Mayo Clinic to use it (see www.healthmanager.mayoclinic.com). You can create profiles for every family member, print questions for doctor's appointments, and receive health guidance information from Mayo Clinic based on your profile. You can also track vital health stats such as blood pressure, weight, and cholesterol that are illustrated in graphs you can share with physicians. Microsoft HealthVault, a platform used by a number of organizations offering PHRs, powers it.

Some PHRs are capable of handling email exchanges between patient and physician, scheduling appointments, and analyzing data uploaded from home monitoring devices such as a blood pressure cuff or heart monitor.

If you are interested in setting up a PHR, first check to see whether the health plan or health-care provider provides one. Why? Because PHRs, according to the American Health Information Management Association, that are not part of a provider's electronic health record are not considered to be legal records and, therefore, are not protected by the same privacy and security protections required of such entities.

On the other hand, a growing number of private companies are offering appealing products. Be sure to carefully review their privacy policies and practices. If you'd like to learn more about PHRs, see what to look for, and view a current listing of PHR companies with links to their websites, go to the American Health Information Management Association website, at www.myphr.com.

Ten questions you should consider when choosing a PHR follow:

1. How will my information be kept private?

2. Are there any circumstances in which my health data would be shared without my permission, and to whom?

3. How can I correct or delete data from my PHR?

4. Can physicians add information to my record?

5. Will I be able to share the PHR with designated family members and my doctor? Can I control what they have access to? Is there a discussion board so we can send emails to each other?

6. Can I upload data from devices such as a blood pressure cuff, home heart monitors, or peak flow monitors? How?

7. What will it cost?

8. Does it have a print feature so I can print information to give to my doctor?

9. Can I import claims data from insurance plans and Medicare?

10. If I change my health plan or the company that I've selected for hosting my PHR goes out of business, what happens to my information?

Organizing your parent's health-care information is a gift that both of you will benefit from many times over.

A Few Pointers on HIPAA Privacy Rules

The Health Insurance Portability and Accountability Act (also known as the HIPAA Privacy Rule) is a law designed to protect an individual's health records from getting into the wrong hands (for example, employers looking for a way to terminate employment or insurance companies trying to find a reason not to provide coverage). It's also intended to allow individuals easier access to their own health records.

As a result of the law, hospitals, doctors, nurses, pharmacies, nursing homes, and other health-care providers have designed ways to make sure that whoever they are giving information to is absolutely legitimate, in an attempt to avoid litigation. Many consumers find the red tape associated with HIPAA to be more trouble than it's worth.

You might have been told that you don't have access to your parent's health status, even in an emergency, like I faced when my mother was being treated for congestive heart failure and I was 2,300 miles away.

I rectified the situation by making sure my mother has a signed HIPAA privacy form allowing me access to her health status and authorizing physicians to speak to me. She's made copies and has a set on the refrigerator in case she needs to hand them to paramedics.

As a caregiver, make sure your parent has signed the appropriate forms giving health-care providers permission to share medical information with you. Upon a hospital admission, they should do the same. Although the law has been around for over a decade, there's still confusion over when family members can be given information about their loved one.

So let's get past the red tape and take a look at examples adapted from the Patient's Guide to the HIPAA Privacy Rule.

- In general, doctors, nurses, and other health-care providers may *not* discuss a patient's past health history or long-term prognosis without specific instructions from that patient.

- An emergency-room doctor may discuss treatment in front of a friend or family member that the patient has invited into the treatment room.

- A doctor may discuss the patient's condition with a parent, spouse, or adult child while the patient is recovering from surgery, emergency care, or other treatment.

- A hospital employee may discuss the patient's bill and questions about it with a family member or friend who is with that patient at the hospital.

- A doctor may speak to someone who is driving the patient home after outpatient surgery, to give instructions to follow on the drive and immediately following your arrival.

- A doctor may discuss drugs prescribed, possible side effects to watch for, and instructions on how to take them with whoever has accompanied the patient during the appointment.

Providers must ask patients for permission, in writing or verbally, or inform them that they are going to discuss the information with a specific person—before they do so. If the patient doesn't object, or if a provider uses his professional judgment to conclude that the patient does not object, he might then proceed. The law does not demand that the patient give permission in writing, but many providers insist on it.

If you're concerned about what will happen if your parent is admitted to the hospital and you are unable to discuss his or her condition, the safest thing is to ask the hospital(s) where your parent will most likely be admitted for a copy of a HIPAA form, and have your parent sign it in advance. You should do the same for every doctor your parent sees. Quite often, your parent will automatically be given these forms at the doctor's office.

If you live far from a parent, it's a good idea to have Mom or Dad sign a letter that identifies your relationship, lists your address and phone number, and gives health-care providers permission to speak to you. Your parent should keep copies available in a conspicuous place so that paramedics called during an emergency can just grab one and give it to emergency-room staff.

Essential Takeaways

- Your parent will likely see a number of specialists, so you need a captain to coordinate all the moving parts of your loved one's care.
- Protect your parents by researching the medications they take, by going to www.medlineplus.com.
- Encourage your parent to use pill tracker containers or electronic dispensers, and maintain a list of all current medications, what each drug is for, who prescribed it, and the dosage.
- Personal health records are an easy, convenient way to organize and share your parent's health-care information among physicians and family members. Just make sure that whatever PHR platform you use ensures security and privacy.

chapter 10

The Insurance Maze

Welcome to the world of Medicare and insurance issues related to older people. No matter how confusing Medicare might feel to you, it's the focal point of your parent's health and is worth whatever effort it takes to navigate it. To their credit, the Centers for Medicare and Medicaid Services have developed a wealth of consumer-friendly materials and a website that can get you any answer you need to know. But a ton of rules and regulations accompany Medicare, so let's discuss the basic parts and the resources available to learn more.

The ABC's and D of Medicare

Medicare is health insurance for people 65 years and older and people who are younger with certain disabilities. It also covers anyone, regardless of age, who suffers from permanent kidney failure that requires dialysis or a kidney transplant known as end-stage renal disease (ESRD).

Medicare has four different parts that cover specific services, classified as Parts A, B, C, and D.

Hospital Insurance: Part A

Medicare covers inpatient care in hospitals, skilled nursing facilities, and hospices. It also covers home health-care services. All those federal Medicare taxes that your parent paid during the working years (40 quarters or more of Medicare-covered employment) have finally paid off with Part A coverage. As a result, few people pay a premium for this coverage. If they don't automatically receive Part A, they should approach Medicare and determine whether they can enroll by paying a premium. However, they do need to meet an annual deductible for inpatient stays. For example, in 2012, the deductible is $1,156 during the first 60 days of an inpatient stay.

Medical Insurance: Part B

Medicare significantly covers physician services, office visits, and other licensed health-care providers, such as physical therapists, respiratory therapists, and occupational therapists. Outpatient care visits, treatments, and procedures are also covered under Part B, including home health care when your parent returns from a hospital stay. For example, if your parent needs physical therapy at home to recover, wheelchairs and other durable medical equipment and supplies are covered under Part B.

Preventive screenings, such as mammograms, prostate tests, colonoscopies, and so on, are covered by Part B. Unlike Part A, your parent needs to pay a Part B premium that Medicare sets every year. It is automatically deducted from Social Security payments and is not increased if there has been no cost of living allowance. For example, in 2012, Medicare Part B premium is $99.90 per month. People with higher annual incomes of above $85,000 (single) and $170,000 (couple) pay more for their premiums. Seniors who have low incomes can receive assistance with their Part B premiums through their state Medical Assistance Medicaid Office.

The level of payment Medicare provides for services under Part B Medical Insurance is usually 80 percent of the cost of the service after an annual deductible ($140 in 2012) has been met. Medicare assigns a set amount for reimbursement to health-care providers. For certain services, there are also co-payments. As a result, most Medicare beneficiaries that participate in "Original Medicare" purchase a health insurance policy to cover the 20 per-cent "gap"—hence, the term *Medigap,* referring to insurance policies sold by private firms to fill in the coverage gap. This type of insurance coverage is explained later in this chapter.

Medicare Advantage Plans: Part C

Beneficiaries can opt to receive Medicare in one of two ways. The first is called "Original Medicare" or "Traditional Medicare." Under this option, beneficiaries can choose their own doctors, and Medicare pays them pre-determined fees for their service, known as assignment. Patients may go to any hospital or physician they want, where and when they want, and Medicare will pay health-care providers directly.

In contrast, opting for a Medicare Advantage Plan essentially means joining a Medicare-approved health maintenance organization (HMO) or preferred provider organization (PPO) run by a private company. Medicare pays these companies a monthly fixed amount for your parent's care. By law, they are required to provide your parent all the services and care he or she would receive from Original Medicare—it must be "equal to or more."

The "advantage" of these plans is that they often provide extra coverage, such as vision care, wellness programs, and, depending on the plan, some dental and hearing coverage. They provide prescription coverage as well (Part D). Those who sign up for an Advantage Plan do not need to pay for a Medigap policy, which can be a sizable savings of close to $300 a month, depending on where you live.

The Medicare Advantage Plans can charge various out-of-pocket costs, such as deductibles and co-pays, and they have their own rules (although these must be approved by Medicare) regarding what doctors beneficiaries must see within their network. Patients continue to pay the Part B pre-mium, and they provide Medicare's services covered under Part A and Part B. The plans set a yearly limit on the amount of out-of-pocket expenses that can be amassed. It's a limit you surely want to explore.

Alert

If your parent has complex needs and has been seeing certain specialists, he or she might want to think twice about joining a Medicare Advantage Plan. Make sure the specialists are in the network—can Mom or Dad accept using the network's physicians, specialists, and hospitals instead of freely finding physicians on his or her own?

Go to www.medicare.gov and click "Compare Drug and Health Plans" to scope out Advantage Plans offered in your area; determine what they cover; and view their deductibles, co-pays, premiums, quality measures, and patient satisfaction ratings.

When searching for a Medicare Advantage Plan provider, here are factors to consider:

- Are your parent's current specialists and primary care doctor in the network?

- Is your parent's favorite hospital in the network?

- Where do patients go for emergencies? Is there a procedure you must follow?

- How easy will it be for your parent to see a specialist? Is a referral required?

- Can your parent change doctors if he or she doesn't like the assigned primary care doctor?

- If your parent lives a few months of the year at a second home or travels, how is he or she covered?

- What skilled nursing homes are in the network?

- What will out-of-pocket expenses be (for example, for prescriptions, doctor visits, hospital stays, or outpatient surgery)?

- What are the monthly premiums, and exactly what do they cover?

One final word of caution: Medicare Health Plans can drop out of the Medicare program any time they want, so look for a plan with a solid financial history. You can refer to A. M. Best's ratings to determine the financial strength and creditworthiness of an insurance company by going to www.ambest.com and clicking on the Consumer section. Remember that your parent can join, switch, or drop a Medicare Advantage Plan during the annual election period, from October 15 through December 7. It's also possible to leave a Medicare Advantage Plan and return to Original Medicare during the Medicare Advantage disenrollment period, from January 1 through February 14. If you choose to go back to Original Medicare, call 1-800-MEDICARE to re-enroll.

Medicare beneficiaries have the opportunity to enroll in Medicare Advantage Plans and Prescription Plans once a year, usually in the fall of the year and lasting for a few months. It's known as the open enrollment period.

Prescription Drug Coverage: Part D

Medicare beneficiaries are offered the opportunity to enroll in a Part D Prescription Plan provided by private companies that Medicare has approved. The beneficiary is responsible for paying a monthly premium and co-pays for the plan. This is a voluntary program; however, those who don't subscribe pay late enrollment penalties if they choose to enroll later. Your parent's premiums will be considerably higher for every year he or she waits.

People with Original Medicare should definitely look for a Part D plan. The costs for premiums, deductibles, and co-pays vary by plan. Beneficiaries who enroll in a Medicare Advantage Plan rarely need to do so, because it's included in the plan. But it's always important to ask before enrolling.

Both plans are affected by what's known as the "donut hole," which is basically a period in which a gap in coverage exists for prescriptions. During this time, your parent would pay nearly all of the prescription costs, up to a limit. However, beneficiaries can get a 50 percent discount on covered brand-name drugs. Between 2011 and 2020, the Affordable Care Act will gradually reduce the share of out-of-pocket expenses, effectively closing the donut hole by 2020.

When you're reviewing plans, be sure to look for any restrictions that might be imposed on drugs your parent takes. Plans categorize drugs into tiers—the higher the tier, the higher the co-pay—or they might require your parent to take a less expensive drug that they deem equivalent. Even if your parent has been in a plan for a year or two, always check during the open enrollment period to see what the plan covers. The plans have formularies—a list of the drugs they cover under their plan. They can decide to change what's on the list from year to year, so if a certain drug is vital to your parent's health, verify that it will continue to be covered.

Comparing Plans

You can compare drug plans offered in your area by going to www. medicare.gov and choosing "Compare Drug and Health Plans." Be sure to have a list handy of all the prescription drugs your parent takes and the pharmacies that fill the prescription. You can also receive extra help to pay for a Part D Plan if you have a limited income. Go to www. benefitscheckup.org to see if you qualify, or contact your state's Medicaid Office.

Medigap Policies: Alphabet Soup

Medigap policies are also known as Medicare Supplement Insurance. This is a private health insurance plan designed to cover health-care costs that Original Medicare does not cover. Quite simply, these plans fill the gap in coverage by supplementing the Original Medicare insurance. Beneficiaries are required to pay for this policy on their own, and your parent should purchase it as soon as he or she is enrolled in Medicare and begins paying Part B premiums.

Every Medigap policy must be approved by Medicare and must follow federal and state laws. The insurance companies offering these plans must sell standardized policies that are identified by the letters A through N—thus, the alphabet soup metaphor. The companies are required to provide the same benefits across the board, per the letter-designated policy they sell.

The letters signify plans that offer different levels of care and service coverage. Less expensive plans, for example, offer fewer benefits, with higher out-of-pocket expenses as a trade-off for paying lower monthly premiums. Medigap policies are sold only to people who have Medicare Part A (Hospital Insurance) and Part B (Medical Insurance). Medicare beneficiaries who are in an Advantage Plan do not need to purchase a Medigap Plan, and insurance companies are prohibited from selling members these unnecessary policies.

Medicaid: State Assistance

Many people confuse Medicaid and Medicare, which is easy to do. They sound somewhat alike, and people mistakenly interchange the names. But they are two very different programs. Medicare, as we've already discussed, is a federal health insurance program for people who are 65 years and older or who are disabled.

Medicaid, by contrast, is a health insurance program administered at the state level for people living at or below the poverty line. The federal government shares the cost with the state. Many older people who qualify for Medicaid are also eligible to receive a federal supplement to their Social Security check, known as SSI.

Medicare is an entitled benefit that is triggered by an age requirement, whereas Medicaid has stringent income eligibility rules and requires an application process. It is meant to provide health coverage for individuals and families who have limited income and resources. Each state has unique eligibility rules on how it calculates income and determines resources.

If your parent qualifies, he or she can receive health-care services from physicians who accept Medicaid, and any hospitalizations and prescriptions would also be covered. If your parent is 65 years or over, he or she would receive Medicare as well—the two are not mutually exclusive. Depending on Mom's or Dad's financial circumstances, Medicaid might cover premiums for Part A and B, along with the deductibles.

Most people start looking at Medicaid when they are facing nursing home costs, which can easily reach $80,000 per year. The state Medicaid program reviews all the "countable income," such as wages, self-employment income, pensions, interest, dividends, annuities, entitlements, and benefits. If the countable income is less than the costs of nursing home care, your parent will likely pass the income test. But he or she also must meet medical requirements that support the need for skilled nursing care in an approved long-term care facility.

You'll often hear the term "spending down" associated with Medicaid and nursing homes. Many people begin paying for a nursing home by using their savings, assets, and income to meet the monthly bill; eventually, they spend their assets down to a level at which they meet federal poverty guidelines. At that point, they apply to Medicaid.

Spending Down

misc.

Years ago, people had to "spend down" to such an extent that the nursing home resident's spouse was impoverished by the time Medicaid helped. But today federal law protects spouses from becoming impoverished. Medical Assistance Offices calculate a monthly Community Spouse Resource Allowance; if the spouse is living in the home, it is not considered a countable asset, nor are the household goods or the car. The state Medicaid office determines the allowance based on an eligibility formula.

Some people think that they can game the system by transferring all of a parent's income and assets to the children as a way of "spending down" so that the parent will immediately qualify for nursing home assistance. You should know, however, that any assets transferred within five years of nursing home admission are *not* exempt from the asset eligibility test. This is often referred to as the "look back" provision.

The Medicaid program also requires repayment of medical assistance for nursing home care from your parent's estate after he or she dies, or from the surviving spouse's estate upon their death. Contact your local welfare office listed in the Blue Pages of your phone book to determine whether your mom would qualify. It might also be wise for you to see a Certified Elder Law Attorney; you can find one in your local area by going to the National Academy of Elder Law Attorneys, at www.naela.org. Chapter 8 provides more information on elder law attorneys.

Today Medicaid offices are redirecting their long-term care dollars for expensive nursing home care to community-based care. So if your parent does qualify for Medicaid, he or she will also be eligible for a wide array of services to help him or her remain in the community rather than be placed in a nursing home.

Long-Term Care Insurance

My mother was one of the first people to sign up for long-term care insurance more than 30 years ago. She had been a nursing home administrator and had become all too familiar with the devastating cost of nursing home care on family finances. Today, at 85 years of age, the policy is providing her home health care and has been a solid return on investment.

Long-term care policies usually offer one or all of the following kinds of care:

- **Nursing home care:** This means skilled nursing care at a long-term care facility. Some nursing homes also provide custodial care and assisted living, which would not be covered under the skilled nursing care provision of the policy. Don't assume that if the care is provided by a nursing home, the care is automatically covered—be sure to ask for clarification. Nursing homes are licensed by the state, and if the facility is Medicare certified, it is also monitored by the federal government. Nursing home care is the major reason most people buy long-term care policies. It's no wonder—people can pay $70,000 to $80,000 a year, depending on where they live.

- **Home health care:** These are services provided at home. They include occupational, physical, respiratory, and speech therapy; nursing care; social work; and nursing assistant services. This is helpful because it gives your parent an alternative to nursing home care.

- **Personal or custodial care:** These services provide help with activities of daily living (ADLs) that are nonmedical, such as assistance with bathing, transfers in and out of beds and chairs, meal preparation, and medication reminders.

- **Respite care:** This is temporary care to relieve a caregiver who provides full-time care to the insured person. For many companies, this is an add-on to a regular policy.

Most companies divide care into three levels:

- Skilled care that requires a doctor's orders and is provided by physicians, nurses, and registered therapists

- Intermediate care that requires trained personnel who are under the supervision of a doctor or nurse

- Custodial care that requires nonmedical personnel to help with the tasks of adult daily living

If your parent lives alone and does not have family members close by, you might want to consider the benefit of custodial care. Dad could be recovering from a bad flu and not need a registered nurse, but he could use someone to cook his meals, shop, get his prescriptions filled, assist with a bath, monitor his health, and alert a family member that he needs to get to the doctor.

In many cases, custodial care can avert a descent down a slippery slope toward frail health and dependency. Make sure the agent clearly spells out what the company defines for each level of care, and have the company tell you who makes care-level decisions.

Most companies require that the person be unable to perform at least two ADL tasks before coverage kicks in (eating, bathing, using the toilet, grooming, and dressing). They frequently send a company nurse to assess the person's condition. Ask the insurance agent about any restrictions surrounding hiring help (for example, whether you can hire a relative who is a nurse's aide). Also ask about the appeal process, in case you disagree with the level-of-care decision made by the company.

Consider compound-inflation rider coverage, which guarantees that the daily benefit amount will increase over time. If your parent buys a policy today that pays out $110 per day, in 20 years, a modest 5 percent inflation rate would generate a nursing home daily rate of $292—nearly three times the amount he or she would receive. With the rider, your premium will cost more, but inflation protection ensures that it's worth what Mom or Dad will really need.

Also be sure the policy is a tax-qualified one. Federal law now allows individuals to deduct a portion of the premium. Check to see whether your parent's state has a 30-day "free look" provision for a long-term care policy so that it can be canceled within 30 days of enrolling if Mom or Dad reconsiders.

Another recommendation is to choose a policy that enables your parent to redirect benefits from home care to nursing home care, and vice versa. For example, if Mom exhausts her nursing home benefit but has untapped home health-care benefits, the company should add the home health-care amount to her nursing home care. Or if she needs to receive care in the home to recover from a hip fracture, for example, it would be helpful to tap into the nursing home benefit.

Look for LTC insurance plans that have been approved by your state as a "Partnership Policy." These plans are available in most states as part of a public-private partnership with the state and insurance companies under the "Long Term Care Partnership Program." The primary advantage is the asset protection provided should all of your benefits be used. The state will disregard assets you own that are equivalent to your policy's benefit limit for purposes of qualifying for Medicaid.

For example, if your policy provides $200,000 worth of benefits and you have depleted the entire $200,000 yet still need long-term care services, Medicaid will disregard $200,000 of personal property/assets for the purposes of qualifying for eligibility. Each state's partnership program requirements are different, so be sure to ask your agent to explain them to you and whether the policy you are considering is a "Partnership Policy."

Policies can be expensive, and the rate increases with age. Long Term Care Quote is a national resource center and independent agency specializing in long-term care insurance that offers easy-to-understand, free comparative quotes to consumers. Visit its website at www.longtermcarequote.com or call them at 1-866-773-0291.

State Health Insurance Programs

Thanks to a federal program known as the State Health Insurance Assistance Program (SHIP), every state in the country offers trained counselors to answer questions regarding health insurance in an objective and easy-to-understand manner. Many states have given their programs a unique name; for example, in Pennsylvania, it is known as the APPRISE Program.

All services are free, and the information is kept confidential. The counselors also provide pamphlets and brochures that explain the benefits and rights under various health insurance programs. SHIP volunteers can help you …

- Decide whether a Medicare Advantage Plan is appropriate for you by explaining the way the network operates compared to Original Medicare.

- Understand your Medicare benefits by explaining what services are covered under Medicare Parts A and B and the Medicare Summary Notice. Medicare mails you that notice every three months to show all your services and supplies billed to Medicare during that period, what Medicare paid, and what you may owe.

- Select a Medigap insurance policy by explaining the benefits offered under each of the standardized insurance plans, and provide a list of companies that sell Medigap insurance policies in your parent's state.

- Obtain assistance to pay for prescription drugs by informing you about government and private programs and signing up for Extra Help with Medicare Part D plans.

- Find government programs that will pay for your parent's Medicare deductibles, co-payments, and Part B premiums, and assist in filling out the paperwork.

- Understand long-term care by explaining which government programs pay for long-term care and reading over the eligibility requirements, and reviewing private long-term care insurance and how to select the best policy.

- Understand all the new options that will be available in the future.

- Process and resolve disputes by being your parent's advocate if Mom or Dad has a problem with Medicare or the Medicare Health Plan provider.

tip

The best way to find your local SHIP program is to call the Eldercare Locator, at 1-800-677-1116. You can also go to www.medicare.gov/contacts, choose the "Search for Specific Organization" option, and then enter "SHIP" on the menu bar.

Fighting Back: Filing Appeals

Chances are, at some point, your parent will be denied a claim for a service, treatment, procedure, or test he or she received from a health-care provider. Don't panic. A good number of times, it's a simple mistake. For example, Medicare uses service codes known as CPT codes to process medical claims. Entering the wrong combination or reversing the numbers can result in denial of the claim. Ask the doctor's office to double-check to make sure it entered the correct code. If not, the office can contact Medicare billing and correct it.

But the answer to the claim denial might not be so simple. If Original Medicare has denied a claim and refuses to pay it, it will send your parent a "Medicare Summary Notice" (MSN). The list includes what it is denying, and you should circle the item(s) that your parent is appealing. Ask the health-care provider who rendered your parent's care to provide a letter or other type of documentation justifying why your parent needed the service. Include a copy of this letter in your appeal.

At the bottom of the MSN, print "Please Review" and then sign the form. Make a copy for your records, include the health-care provider's letter, and mail the MSN to the address specified within 120 days of receiving the denial notice. Even if your parent has signed an Advance Beneficiary Notice (ABN) stating that he or she would pay for the care if Medicare decides not to, you still can appeal and should. According to the Center for Medicare Rights, 80 percent of Medicare Part A (Hospital) appeals turn out favorably for the beneficiary, and 92 percent of Part B (Doctors & Outpatient Services) do so.

Appeals Process for Medicare Advantage Plans

If your parent belongs in one of these plans and not Original Medicare, look over the plan's handbook describing appeal rights, which are somewhat different from Original Medicare. For example, beneficiaries have only 60 days from the date of a denial notice to file an appeal, which is half the length of time allowed with Original Medicare.

Now what about that ABN your parent signed? ABNs are meant to protect consumers from unexpected financial liability in cases when Medicare will likely deny payment. An ABN gives beneficiaries the opportunity to decide whether they want to still receive the service (this also applies to medical supplies and equipment).

If your parent receives an ABN from a doctor or health-care provider, absolutely take the time to read it. Together you can then decide, for example, whether to find another doctor or health-care provider who will provide the service and can meet the eligibility guidelines set by Medicare to have the service covered.

According to the Centers for Medicare and Medicaid Services, if a consumer receives an ABN, he or she should choose one of two options on the form:

- **Option 1:** Checking this option indicates that a person does want to receive the service or item and that the claim will be sent to Medicare. Your parent might be billed while Medicare is making its decision. If Medicare pays, your mom or dad will be refunded any payments due to them. But if Medicare denies payment, your parent will be personally and fully responsible for payment. Your parent will have the right to appeal Medicare's decision. Medicare will not decide whether to pay unless you receive the service or item and have a claim submitted.

- **Option 2:** Choosing this option indicates that a person does not want to receive the service or item, and a claim will not be sent to Medicare. Your parent will not be able to appeal the supplier's, physician's, or provider's opinion that Medicare won't pay.

In other words, the only way to appeal the decision is to chance it and say "Yes" on the ABN form. Medicare needs an actual claim for services in order to deny it. If you don't want to take the risk, seek second opinions from other physicians and providers to see whether they can meet your needs and the eligibility requirements of Medicare.

Remember, the appeal rate for favorable outcomes for beneficiaries is very high, so it might be worth the risk. But only you and your parent can make this decision.

Tip

Fiscal intermediaries are private companies that contract with The Centers for Medicare and Medicaid Services to pay Medicare Part A and B bills (for example, hospital, skilled nursing care, and physician services). If you have a dispute or need further information on a claim or denial, contact the company phone number that appears on the Explanation of Benefits or Medicare Summary Notice. You can also call Medicare at 1-800-Medicare to find a fiscal intermediary.

When dealing with any kind of insurance denial, take these steps:

- Ask for a written explanation of why the claim was denied. Most state laws require companies to do so, but if you don't receive it, demand it.

- Maintain thorough records. When you talk to a claim's representative on the phone, write down his or her name and make notes of what was said; keep copies of all correspondence from the rep and you. If you don't hear back, send another letter with a copy of your original. Always cite your policy number on your correspondence.

- Before you file an appeal, look up your plan's requirements and steps to file a proper appeal so that you don't lose time in the process. And don't accept the company telling you that the reason your appeal was denied is that you incorrectly filled out the form or filed late. If the service was properly given and is covered under your insurance, you have a right to pursue its coverage.

- Approach the doctor or other health-care provider to help your cause. Show the denial letter and relevant language from your policy so the office knows how to respond to the denial letter. Include it in your appeal.

- Ask to see the report issued by the findings of the insurance company's medical advisors. The reviewers should be experts in the field relevant to the surgery, procedure, or service that you were denied. If not, ask for a medical opinion from such an expert.

A terrific resource for understanding your Medicare rights, steps to take, and resources is offered by the Center for Medicare Rights (www.medicarerights.org), a nonprofit organization dedicated to ensuring that beneficiaries receive what they deserve. The Center has a Medicare Interactive feature in which you enter your question or topic and get an answer and links to additional information. You can go directly to this service at www.medicareinteractive.org or call the helpline at 1-800-333-4114.

If you need professional help beyond what a SHIP volunteer can offer, private companies can assist. Health Proponent (www.healthproponent.com) provides an initial consultation for a $29.95 annual membership fee and then charges additional fees, depending on what's required. It can negotiate a reduction in the insurance bill, in return for a percentage of the savings. Call 1-866-939-3435 for more.

What's the bottom line? Always question a bill that you think Medicare and/or your parent's insurance company should have covered. Far too often, conscientious, bill-paying elderly don't question their doctor's office or hospital bills and simply pay. Some even fear that they might be refused further treatment if they appeal or question the bill. That just isn't so. The fiscal intermediaries are paid by Medicare to resolve these issues—so make use of the service.

Essential Takeaways

- Medicare is the bedrock of your parent's health care, and two options are available: Original Medicare and Medicare Advantage plans.

- Medicare beneficiaries in Original Medicare should also carry a Medigap insurance policy that covers the gap in coverage between what Medicare will pay (assigns) a provider and what the provider actually charges.

- Long-term care insurance can be helpful in protecting older people's assets in case they ever need nursing home care. It's wise to purchase plans with inflation protection and those that allow the elderly to interchange coverage between nursing home and home health-care benefits.

- It's always worth the effort to appeal a denied claim, whether by Medicare or another insurance carrier. Reach out to your health-care provider to assist you with justification for the service received. SHIP volunteers in your state are a great resource.

chapter 11

When Your Parent Is Hospitalized

Planning ahead for an admission

Making sense of the world of hospitals

Standing guard against medical errors

Fighting back an early discharge

Interpreting the foreign language of medical terms

It's bound to happen. If you're caring for anyone 70 years and up, chances are good that he or she will land in the hospital sooner or later. A fall in the bathroom, a medication mix-up, a seriously bad case of the flu, or an appointment with a surgeon's knife can throw both of you into a tailspin. Caught off guard with serious decisions to make, families can quickly find themselves disagreeing on what to do—or they simply can't make any decisions.

Stay in control and avoid the squabbling by learning what to ask, who to talk to, how to stay clear of medical errors, and how to advocate for your loved one.

The First Hurdle: Finding the Best Hospital

Most of us live in communities that have several hospitals. But we rarely think of shopping around for one like we do for schools or a bank. Many times the choice is made for us because a surgeon or doctor has an affiliation with the hospital. But in today's networked world, many physicians work with multiple hospitals. Depending on why your loved one is being admitted, one hospital might be a far better choice than another.

So why does comparing hospitals matter, and how can you know? Hospitals are faced with hard economic choices, just like all businesses. They can't possibly afford every piece of break-through medical equipment in every single specialty. Nor can they afford unlimited staff, so they steer their resources toward areas where they'll get their best return on investment. The trick is to make sure that their "best return" is your best interest. If you are worried about a stroke, find a hospital specializing in treating brain attacks described in Chapter 1. For a heart condition, go to the hospital with the best open-heart surgery recovery rates. If Mom or Dad is at high risk for emergency department visits, find a hospital with a specialized geriatric emergency room.

If you've ever used *Consumer Reports* to decide on what computer, television, or appliance to buy, you'll find the Hospital Compare feature by the Centers for Medicare and Medicaid (CMS) similar in ease of use and chock full of solid information. You can learn how hospitals perform in treating heart attacks, heart failure, and pneumonia, and how patients recover from common surgeries under their care. The site even posts mortality rates for key conditions within 30 days of patients being hospitalized.

If you like reading about other people's experiences, such as at restaurants or hotels, you'll especially like CMS survey results on patients' hospital experiences. Among 28 questions, patients report on whether their pain was controlled, whether nurses and doctors explained things in a way they could understand, and how long they waited for a call button to be answered.

So if your family is in a quandary about which hospital is best for your loved one, get the facts.

Tip

Compare how your local hospitals perform by going to the Centers for Medicare and Medicaid (CMS) website at www.hospitalcompare.hhs.gov. Don't have the internet? Then call Medicare at 1-800-633-4227, say "Other choices" at the end of the menu options, and then ask for an agent to give you hospital comparison information.

Once Admitted, Are You Really a Patient?

During a winter trip to Florida, 76-year-old Ruth exhibited the classic signs of a stroke: her right arm and hand went numb, and her speech became slurred. Two days before that, her retinal specialist had alerted her that the plaques in her right eye could foreshadow a potential stroke. So Ruth wasted no time in getting to the emergency room. The doctors diagnosed a *transient ischemic attack* (*TIA*).

A **transient ischemic attack (TIA)** exhibits symptoms similar to a stroke or brain attack, but it generally lasts only a few minutes and causes no permanent damage. It is caused by a blockage of blood to the brain. A TIA is often called a "mini stroke," but it shouldn't be ignored: about one in three people who have a TIA eventually suffers a stroke, and about half strike within a year after the TIA.

Given her mother's history of strokes and the danger of TIAs often preceding a stroke, she was admitted to the hospital. Ruth spent three days in her hospital room undergoing tests, wearing a nifty hospital gown, and receiving the care that patients receive. But a few months later, Medicare sent her a walloping bill—she was never an "inpatient."

So what happened? Did Ruth not act like a patient? Did they get her Medicare ID mixed up? It turns out that Medicare now has two ways of classifying people admitted to hospitals: inpatients and those receiving "observational care." Ruth's physician admitted her under observation, so despite the fact that she was admitted to the hospital as a patient (sure sounds like inpatient), her observational status meant that Medicare would not cover any of the prescriptions she was given over those three days. The bill ran into the thousands of dollars.

Being under observational status also meant that Medicare would not cover any rehabilitation care for Ruth in a skilled nursing facility if she needed it. Why? Medicare pays only for care in a skilled nursing facility when a patient has spent at least three consecutive days (not including the day of discharge) in a hospital before being admitted to a nursing home. In this instance, Medicare might pay up to 100 days of rehabilitation and skilled nursing care. But if those three days are under observation, as in Ruth's case, they don't meet Medicare's "three hospital days" criteria to trigger skilled nursing care coverage. And that price tag can run into the tens of thousands! As of 2012, Congress was considering rescinding this rule, but no action has been taken. Check my website (www.lindarhodescaregiving. com) for updates.

Bottom line? Don't expect that someone will tell you whether your loved one has been admitted to the hospital as an "inpatient" or under "observational care." Ask the doctor. If you've been told your parent is under "observational status," ask to speak to a social worker or patient advocate to find out why, what you will be expected to pay, and what you can do to appeal the decision.

Alert

Experts and consumer advocates expect that the use of observational status by hospitals will escalate as Medicare slaps fines on hospitals for inappropriate patient readmissions. In Medicare's view, this signals inadequate patient care while they were in the hospital. So hospitals will reduce their exposure to readmission penalties by placing more patients on observational status.

If your loved one is labeled "observational," the Center for Medicare Advocacy and other consumer groups recommend these steps:

1. Contact your personal physician and ask him or her to call the hospital to request a change in status. Be aware, however, that your doctor cannot over rule the hospital.

2. Ask the hospital to provide you notice (Advance Beneficiary Notice) in writing of your level of care and why.

3. If you enter a skilled nursing facility after discharge from the hospital, ask the nursing facility to bill Medicare. If Medicare denies the claim because you did not meet the three-day rule due to observational status, appeal it. Call Medicare at 1-800-633-4227 for more information.

4. If the nursing home won't bill Medicare, complete a "Notice of Exclusions from Medicare Benefits: Skilled Nursing Facility" form and ask the facility to submit it to Medicare so you can get an official decision on your coverage (or lack of it). When you get the decision, if it is not in your favor, appeal it.

5. If your parent has been discharged from the hospital to nursing home care, be sure to review the Medicare Summary Notice explanation of benefits to see whether coverage has been limited due to observational status. Appeal to the Medicare billing contractor; if it's denied, appeal again.

For an overview of inpatient and observation care from Medicare, read the brochure, "Are you a Hospital Inpatient or Outpatient?" You can find this on my website, www.lindarhodescaregiving.com. Click the *Caregiving Without Conflict* book cover.

Meet the Hospitalist

Long gone are the days of Marcus Welby, MD, coming to see you in the hospital. Today you're greeted by a crowd of specialists, technicians, therapists, and nurses. With so many older people suffering from multiple chronic conditions—diabetes, arthritis, and high or low blood pressure—different specialists are called in to monitor each part of their care. Let's say that your mother is admitted to the hospital for hip surgery, but during the course of her stay, her blood pressure skyrockets and her blood sugar plummets. Neither of these conditions will be treated by the orthopedic surgeon.

So who decides to do what? A relatively new type of doctor—the hospitalist. This physician oversees a patient's care from start to finish during the entire hospital stay. He or she orders tests, coordinates treatment plans with other specialists, prescribes medications, consults with the primary care doctor, and arranges for discharge. Most hospitalists are internists, and they know how to work the hospital's system on a patient's behalf. Their mission is to get the entire medical team on the same page and ensure that no patient falls through the cracks. The good thing is that most medical errors take place during the classic hand-off.

The hospitalist interacts with family members and patients more than the other specialists. If you have questions about your loved one's care, ask for the hospitalist. Tracking him or her down will be much easier than trying to catch a surgeon during early morning rounds. The hospitalist can also take the time to explain the many moving parts of your loved one's care.

Tip

Before meeting with a hospitalist, be sure to write down your questions and ask other family members whether they have any questions they would like you to ask. Don't be afraid to ask the doctor to show you pictures or other illustrations that will help explain what's going on with your loved one. Be sure to share the information with other family members so that they, too, are on the same page and feel included.

Here is what you should ask to make sure that both the hospitalist and your primary care doctor are talking.

What to ask the primary care doctor:

- What procedures does your practice have in place to coordinate my parent's care with a hospitalist?

- How soon does the hospitalist contact you to let you know my parent has been admitted to the hospital?

- How often do you talk to the hospitalist while my parent is in the hospital? Is there a daily update, or does the hospitalist call only if there is a problem?

- Does the hospitalist know how to reach you?

- What information do you share with the hospitalist?

- Will you let him or her know about my parent's medical history, prescriptions, and allergies?

- Does the hospitalist send you a copy of my parent's discharge summary and test results? How soon?

- Will your office call my parent to set up a follow-up visit when discharged, or does my parent call you?

What to ask the hospitalist (first, find out who the hospitalist is):

- Have you informed my parent's primary care doctor that he or she has been admitted?

- Have you received my parent's medical history from his or her primary care doctor?

- Is there anything else you need to know?

- How often do you plan to speak to my parent's physician while admitted to the hospital here?

- Upon discharge, ask: Have you sent my parent's discharge summary and test results to his or her primary care doctor?

- If I or my parent has any questions about discharge directions, should we call you or my parent's physician?

When it's time for your loved one to leave the hospital, ask the hospitalist if your parent's discharge summary and test results are being sent to your parent's primary physician. If not, ask the hospitalist to send them. Your parent needs this information in their medical records for follow-up visits.

Getting Out Alive

I once met with a team of physicians at a large urban medical center to discuss the high rate of medical errors taking place in hospitals. At the end of the meeting, I asked them what one piece of advice they'd give my readers on how to remain safe in a hospital. One doctor promptly quipped, "Don't come."

He went on to say that patients can do a lot to stay clear of hospitals: don't smoke, lose weight, eat healthy, exercise, and take required medications that maintain health. In other words, he felt patients were partly to blame for placing themselves at risk of being hospitalized in the first place.

But that's certainly not the whole story. Sometimes we absolutely require the care that's provided only at a hospital. Under those circumstances, we need everyone at that hospital to be accountable. But startling statistics tell us otherwise. Every month, one in seven hospitalized Medicare patients suffers at least one "adverse event" due to a medical error. According to the Office of Inspector General (OIG) of the Department of Health and Human Services, 134,000 people a month, or 1.6 million a year, become victims of medical mistakes. Tragically, 15,000 people a month, amassing to an astounding 180,000 people a year, die as a result of those errors.

What are those adverse events? According to the OIG, they include infections from surgery and catheters, incorrect dose of a drug, severe bed sores, inadequate wound care, patient falls, IV fluids given incorrectly, equipment failure, and the sensationalized surgical mistakes we've all read about when a surgeon has operated on the wrong patient or wrong body part.

So now that I have your attention, follow these steps to prevent your loved one from becoming one of those adverse events:

- Be at your loved one's bedside as much as possible, especially during the first few days after surgery. You can speak up for him or her, observe symptoms to tell the nurse, and make sure the call button is being answered.

- Question whether a catheter is absolutely necessary, because they increase the risk of bladder and kidney infections. If one is required, ask whether it's still needed every few days, just to make sure no one has forgotten to remove it.

- Anyone who enters the room and intends to touch your loved one should wash his or her hands in front of you, put on new gloves, or use an alcohol gel. If anyone hasn't, ask him or her to do so. Hospital-acquired infections are lethal and are readily passed to patients from doctors, nurses, and aides who've touched an infected patient.

- If your loved one has a wound, keep an eye out for dressings that haven't been changed, have become loose, or emit a foul odor.

- Elderly patients have fragile skin. If they are confined to a bed for a few days, a small red sore on bony areas such as knees, heels, elbows, and buttocks can turn into a gaping wound. Make sure your loved on is on an airflow mattress and is being repositioned every two hours.

One of the most feared complications following surgery or from being confined to a bed for prolonged periods is the formation of a blood clot. These form in leg veins, known as DVT (deep venous thrombosis), causing pain, redness, and swelling. If the blood clot breaks off, travels, and lodges itself in a lung, a pulmonary embolus occurs and can cause respiratory failure.

Ask the doctor what steps he or she is taking to make sure your loved one won't develop a blood clot. Three of the most common treatment strategies are heparin (blood thinner) injections, pneumatic boots that continuously inflate and deflate around the calves of the legs, and efforts to start walking as soon as possible.

Following my father's surgery, an aide helped him with his first walk down the hall, and I accompanied her. Something just didn't seem right about my father. He appeared pale and troubled. She asked him if he was okay, and he said "Sure" and kept walking. But I told her something was wrong and felt that he should go back to bed and she should get the doctor. Once in bed, this World War II veteran told me he didn't want to appear like a "sissy" and felt he should tough it out and keep walking. He ended up in the intensive care unit; the doctor diagnosed him with a pulmonary embolus.

How to Stop an Early Discharge

Giving you advice on how to stay longer in the hospital might seem ironic—we just talked about reasons you shouldn't want to be there in the first place.

But hospital care can also do absolute wonders. Lives are made better, families take home loved ones who were at death's door, and health is restored. Asking patients to leave the hospital's cocoon of comprehensive care before they're ready can undo all that's been accomplished. It doesn't take much to unravel an elderly person's fragile health.

From the moment your loved one has been admitted, a discharge planner has been monitoring his or her care and projecting a departure date. Nothing like, "Here's your hat, what's your hurry," right? But Medicare does require that a patient's discharge from the hospital be "safe and adequate."

Sending someone home alone or into a situation where he or she will not receive adequate care (because, for instance, he or she lives alone or has a spouse with significant health problems) is not considered a safe discharge. Be sure to let the physician and discharge planners know of your parent's circumstances.

If you think your loved one is being discharged too soon, talk with the doctor first to see whether he or she can change the discharge date. If not, you have the right to appeal. Here are the steps to follow:

1. Contact the Quality Improvement Organization (QIO) no later than the planned discharge date. The QIO is an outside reviewer hired by Medicare to assess your loved one's case and determine whether he or she is ready to leave the hospital. You should have received the QIO's contact information at admission, along with "An Important Message from Medicare About Your Rights."

2. You can contact the QIO any day of the week. Once you speak to someone or leave a message, your appeal has begun.

3. You will receive a notice from the hospital or Medicare Managed Care plan (if you belong to one) explaining why it has decided to discharge your loved one.

4. The QIO will then ask for your opinion. You or your loved one can talk with the representative or submit a written statement.

5. The QIO will review all the information and medical records regarding your case, and it will notify you of its decision one day after it has received all the necessary information to review it.

6. If the QIO determines that your loved one is not ready for discharge, Medicare will continue to cover the services. If it disagrees, Medicare will continue to cover the services until noon of the day *after* the QIO notified you of its decision.

Once you make the appeal, your care is covered while the QIO is reviewing the case. Some social workers have told me that this can gain up to two days in the hospital while the case is being reviewed. Remember, even if the QIO decides that the discharge is valid, your hospital stay will be covered during the time it took to review the case and up to noon of the day following its notification to you of the decision.

You should also know that Medicare provides appeal rights for other health-care providers, too. These are skilled nursing facilities (nursing homes), home health agencies, comprehensive outpatient rehabilitation centers, and hospice.

So if you believe that your loved one isn't ready to go or the discharge isn't safe, make the call.

Everybody's Favorite: Emergency Rooms

Well, first off, we're not supposed to call them "emergency rooms" any longer (good thing the hit television show *ER* is off the air). They are "emergency departments," which makes a lot more sense, given the sophisticated action that takes place amid a slew of trauma rooms, triage stations, and exam rooms.

> **Alert**
>
> In light of how disorienting the fast pace of trauma care can be for the elderly, some hospitals have created geriatric emergency rooms that specialize in the urgent care of seniors. Geriatricians familiar with multiple chronic conditions of older patients and the wide range of drugs many of them take are adept at quickly assessing what's wrong and treating the unique needs of the aging body.

No one really wants to go to an emergency department. The long waits are notorious, yet if they take you immediately, you know you must be in real trouble. Fainting from the pain of a kidney stone got me through triage in a matter of minutes. But I sure don't recommend trying this "stunt" to shorten your wait.

Hopefully, the care your loved one receives in the emergency department will render him or her well enough to go home and recover. If not, you might need to convince a physician to admit your loved one to the hospital. Consider my mother's story.

My 84-year-old mother broke her shoulder and left leg in a fall and had just been admitted to a skilled rehabilitation facility. When I came in the next morning, she confided, "They almost dropped me in the bathroom." At bedtime following another shaky transfer, she started to complain of pains near her chest and her blood pressure was very elevated. Wondering whether she had a broken rib or her congestive heart failure was acting up, I called 911.

The emergency department physician ran cardiovascular tests and felt confident that her heart was fine, but he wasn't 100 percent sure. He diagnosed that her chest wall had suffered soft tissue damage from being poorly handled. Still, he told me that she was good to go.

Go to what? There was no way on God's green earth that I was taking her back to the facility that had just injured her—while, by the way, I watched five staff members take a 30-minute break while call lights went unanswered.

I pleaded with him. "But her orthopedic doctor wrote an order that she needs two people to transfer her, she's legally blind due to macular degeneration, she breaks her fragile osteoarthritic bones (this was her third in as many months), she has a cast on her right side, she has a soft tissue injury, she's wearing a cast up to her groin on her left side, and she's also exhibiting signs of gout. Doesn't all this count for something? Isn't there some way you can admit her?" But he apologetically explained that Medicare is much more aggressive about denying hospital claims, and hospital utilization review committees are reversing doctor's orders to admit. He warned me that, if he did admit her, she could be picking up the tab. We said that we'd take the risk for one day. He asked for a little more time to review Medicare criteria given the additional medical information I provided. My mother was subsequently admitted.

A day later, the hospital review committee agreed and allowed her to stay in the hospital for three days to receive the level of care she needed. The inpatient hospital stay enabled her to be transferred to a subacute rehab facility that met her rather complicated needs for a six-week recovery—and Medicare did cover it. But if I hadn't spoken up, I would have been taking my mother back home in an ambulance, and for the life of me, I didn't know how I could have cared for her by myself or afforded 24-hour home health care that would have required two people for six weeks. Learn to speak up!

What Are They Saying? Understanding Medicalese

You have a right to ask doctors and nurses to explain to you the diagnosis and treatment of your loved one. All too often, older people think that asking too many questions might come off as rude or that they might appear stupid in front of the doctor. So they dutifully nod like they understand. In some cases, that pretense can get them into a lot of trouble with their health.

The best decisions are informed decisions. As consumers, we need to educate ourselves, at least on the basics of our health conditions and the treatments that doctors might prescribe for our recovery. In Chapter 1, I showed you how to research medical conditions and formulate questions to ask your doctor and other specialists. But right now, I'd like to share my Medicalese Decoder so you understand the foreign language spoken in hospital country. Feel free to get an electronic copy to print at my website, at www.lindarhodescaregiving.com. Just click the "Caregiver Tips" section.

Before you review the following terms, take a moment to understand the pattern used to create them. Basically, each term is made up of a root word plus a suffix. Breaking the term into these two parts can help you better decode its meaning.

The "root" word is the object of the ailment—the body part, for example. The suffix is the ending of the word and refers to some aspect of the root term. For example, the suffix *pathy* means "disease." So when you see a word ending in *pathy,* it's referring to a disease, as in *nephropathy,* which means "disease of the kidney" (nephro). There are a number of suffixes or endings to medical terms that simply mean "pertaining to": *-ac, -al, -ary, -ic, -ical, -ous, -tic,* and *-ar.* For example, *cardiac* means "pertaining to the heart," *venous* means "pertaining to the vein," and *pelvic* means "pertaining to the pelvis."

With this background information in mind, here's my Medicalese Decoder of common medical terms:

Medicalese Decoder for Body Parts

Root Word for Body Parts	What It Means	Example
Cardi	Heart	Cardiac arrest (heart stopping)
Coli	Large intestine or colon	Colitis (inflammation of the colon)

Root Word for Body Parts	What It Means	Example
Derm	Skin	Dermatologist (doctor specializing in skin)
Duodeno	Small intestine	Duodenum (first part of the small intestine)
Encephal	Brain	Encephalitis (inflammation of the brain)
Gastro	Stomach	Gastroenteritis (stomach flu)
Hemo/a	Blood	Hemodialysis (dialysis machine that filters waste products from the blood)
Hepat	Liver	Hepatitis (inflammation of the liver)
Myel	Spinal cord or bone marrow	Myelofibrosis (disorder of the bone marrow)
Nephro	Kidney	Nephropathy (damage or disease of the kidney)
Neur	Nerves	Neurotoxin (a substance that damages nerves)
Opthal or ocul	Eye	Ophthalmologist (eye doctor)
Oste	Bone	Osteoporosis (bones that become porous, making them fragile)
Phleb or ven	Vein	Intravenous (within a vein, such as with IV therapy)
Pneumo	Lung	Pneumonia (infection of the lung)

Medicalese Decoder for Conditions

Suffix for Conditions	What It Means	Example
-algia	Pain	Myalgia (muscle pain)
-itis	Inflammation	Cervicitis (inflammation of the cervix)
-lith	Stones or calcifications	Tonsillolith (tonsil stone)
-oid	Resembles	Fibroid (noncancerous tumor of connective tissue)

Suffix for Conditions	What It Means	Example
-oma	Tumor	Lymphoma (cancer in lymphatic cells, affecting the immune system)
-pathy	Disease	Nephropathy (disease of the kidney)
-phasia	Speech	Aphasia (without speech, usually following a stroke)
-plegia	Paralysis	Hemiplegia (paralysis affecting only one side of the body)
-rrhage	Burst forth	Hemorrhage (blood escaping from blood vessels)
-sclerosis	Hardening	Atherosclerosis (thickening of the artery wall)

Medicalese Decoder for Surgeries and Procedures

Suffix for Surgery and Procedures	What It Means	Example
-centesis	Tap or puncture to drain fluid	Amniocentesis (drawing fluid from the amniotic sac)
-ectomy	Removal of	Mastectomy (surgical removal of one or both breasts)
-oscopy	To examine with a scope to explore the body cavity	Colonoscopy (examination of the colon)
-ostomy	Small surgical hole leading out of the body	Tracheostomy (incision in the trachea)
-otomy	Large surgical opening	Ovariotomy (surgical incision of an ovary)
-tripsy	To crush	Lithotripsy (procedure to crush kidney stones)

Don't be afraid to ask a doctor or nurse to spell out any term you don't understand—and the same with medications. Without the correct spelling, you won't be able to properly use the Medicalese Decoder.

Here's hoping for a safe, nurturing, and restorative hospital stay!

Essential Takeaways

- Become your loved one's patient advocate by planning ahead, learning what questions to ask, and remaining by his or her bedside.

- Don't be intimidated by all the white coats and fancy titles. You have every right to ask questions and expect answers that anyone can understand.

- Hospital care can be a lifesaver, but it can take lives, too. Just remember that you're not powerless: hand-washing practices, pertinent questions, bedsore prevention, adequate wound dressings, and catheter management are all issues under your control.

- You don't have to take no for an answer. You can appeal a hospital's decision to discharge your loved one when you believe it's not safe for him or her to leave.

- Learn to use the Medicalese Decoder of common medical terms to help you better understand the language hospitals and medical professionals use.

chapter 12

End-of-Life Care

Working through a life-ending diagnosis

Getting everyone on the same page with an advance directive

Understanding the needs of a dying person

Managing the pain through palliative care

Making the hospice decision

The irony of dying is that, even though death is a solo act, the process of getting there and the final moments surrounding it are anything but solitary. Family members, even those who might be estranged, become intensely involved. Each bring their own view on death and struggle with the process of dying within themselves and with others. Everyone, including the person dying, also interacts with a group of strangers: nurses, doctors, therapists, and social workers. The conversations and topics are intimate, but the decisions made are in many ways quite public.

None of us is truly prepared for what we'll feel and do when a loved one is given a life-ending diagnosis. Even the life of a centenarian feels short when the one you love is an integral part of your life. But it does help to know what to expect from health-care professionals, what makes a "good death," and how to navigate your own emotional journey. And that's what this chapter addresses.

Stages of Coming to Terms with the End of Life

Perhaps the most well-known description of what people feel when they are confronted with a life-ending illness comes from psychiatrist Elizabeth Kübler-Ross. In her groundbreaking book, *On Death and Dying,* she introduced what is now known as the Five Stages of the Grief Cycle or the Five Stages of Loss. Grief is also a psychological response to other emotional trauma, such as a divorce, loss of a job, or a major catastrophe such as 9/11.

You, your parent, your siblings, and your close relatives might go through one or all of these stages, and you'll surely go through them at your own pace. Kübler-Ross never meant for the stages to be taken literally. We don't go through them step by step or in the order she presents them. Some of us move in and out of various stages, some remain trapped in one stage, others revisit certain stages, and some might skip various stages altogether.

But all in all, her model provides a worthy guide based on years of study and experience that might help you better understand and appreciate the barrage of emotions coming your way.

Kübler-Ross's model is sometimes referred to by the acronym DABDA, standing for denial, anger, bargaining, depression, and acceptance. According to her stages, here's how emotions play out when coping with grief:

Denial: "I'm okay. This really isn't happening to me." Denial is a natural reaction to information that's catastrophic and life changing. It's the mind's buffer to a terrible reality, allowing you a timeout and a chance to regroup. Because you can't escape the reality when it comes to dying and death, denial serves as a temporary defense against an impending crisis.

Anger: "Why me? It's just not fair!" By the mere act of asking this question, it's apparent that an individual is no longer in denial. But the reality makes the person angry, volatile, and upset. The person may displace his or her anger by finding fault with others, may act out against any form of treatment, or they might turn inward and blame him- or herself. You'll need to be understanding and allow your loved one to vent this anger without taking it personally. It's a trying stage for everyone.

Bargaining: "If I make amends or do something good, maybe I can buy more time." It starts with an internal conversation between oneself and whomever that person believes to be God or a higher power. The person hopes that if he or she takes certain favorable actions, the reward will be more time or the ability to beat the odds of dying altogether. It's not uncommon for the bargaining to be linked with surviving long enough to attend a significant life event, such as a daughter's wedding, the birth of a grandchild, or the completion of a major project.

Depression: "I'm so incredibly sad. Why go on?" During this fourth stage, the dying person begins mourning his or her own death and the loss of all he or she would have known. Some experts refer to this as "anticipatory grief." Regret, fear, crying, and wanting to be alone are all psychological responses that can be expected. It is a heartbreaking, necessary process and not something you can simply treat with cheerful encouragement.

Acceptance: "It's my time, and I'm okay with it." This stage is expressed in as many ways as there are fingerprints, but underneath it all is a deep sense of having come to terms with one's mortality. For some, it may take the form of a sense of peace and calm, whereas others view it as their fate and see no reason to fight it. It's not unusual for the dying person to reach this stage before his or her family members do. As a result, it may appear to those who are still struggling that their loved one has become emotionally detached.

It's no wonder such a daunting, life-changing event runs the gamut of emotions and why it's so unlikely that you, your parent, your siblings, and other loved ones will be on the same page throughout it. Be patient with each other. If someone is angry, let him or her express those feelings without taking it personally. If another person is in denial, let him or her remain in this "unrealistic" cocoon until he or she is ready to cope with the harsh reality that lies ahead. Grieving is natural; don't suffocate it by avoiding the sadness and pain that comes with loss.

The grieving process is an emotionally charged roller-coaster ride, and there's no such thing as closure. But as you can see in the following story about my brother, if you focus on your loved one's needs and let that guide you, you and your family should be okay.

My youngest brother was only 44 years old when he was told he had stage IV malignant melanoma. It came out of the blue; his only symptom had been an upset stomach that his doctor had attributed to a possible ulcer. But then one day he lost his vision for about 10 minutes in his right eye. A CT scan of his brain, lungs, and liver rendered the horrible verdict. Within 12 weeks, my brother was gone.

Our family experienced all the stages I've just described. We went through them both alone and together. Some of us were more angry than others. We'd go in and out of denial depending on which doctor talked to us. We desperately searched the internet for clinical trials. I watched my mother hide in a restaurant's bathroom sobbing while we celebrated Mother's Day, knowing it was her "baby's" last.

My brother did reach the stage of acceptance. He told me one day that this simply was his fate, and he was at peace with it. His greatest regret was not being able to raise his young children, but he knew we'd all band together as a family and look out for them. From that point on, he became more spiritual. He made his own funeral arrangements and gave us each special gifts to show how much he loved and appreciated us. He reached into the future and bought each child a piece of jewelry to be given to them when they graduated from high school.

Seventy percent of Americans do not have a living will, also known as an advance directive, that describes their end-of-life care wishes. It's a document that can save a lot of second-guessing under dire circumstances. Let's take a look at what these are and how to do one.

Living Wills or Advance Directive

Living wills, also known as advance directives, focus on end-of-life decisions and enable you to express your wishes about medical care in case you face a life-ending condition or enter a state of permanent unconsciousness and can no longer make your own medical decisions. The living will takes effect when a doctor determines that death is fairly certain or that the person is in a persistent state of unconsciousness. The living will directs a physician to withhold or withdraw life-sustaining treatment that serves only to prolong the process of dying. However, the directive also states what measures should be taken to provide comfort and relieve pain. Most living will documents state whether the individual does or does not want any of the following forms of treatment:

- Cardiac resuscitation

- Mechanical respiration

- Tube feeding or any other artificial or invasive form of nutrition (food) or hydration (water)

- Blood or blood products

- Any form of surgery or invasive diagnostic tests

- Kidney dialysis

- Antibiotics

The living will declaration becomes effective when your doctor receives a copy of it and determines that you are incompetent and in a terminal condition or a state of permanent unconsciousness. In most states, you must sign the document in front of two witnesses who are 18 or older.

Tip	Aging with Dignity offers an excellent "Five Wishes" living will that is very complete and helpful. It takes you through common-sense questions to help you make end-of-life care decisions. Order a copy at www. agingwithdignity.org or call 1-888-5WISHES (1-888-594-7437). Many hospitals also offer copies of living wills upon admission. The living will does not have to be notarized or executed by a lawyer. Be sure to give copies of it to physicians and the hospital.

In some states, a living will is not effective in the event of a medical emergency that involves ambulance personnel; paramedics are required to perform CPR unless they are given separate orders that state otherwise. These orders are commonly referred to as "nonhospital do-not-resuscitate orders" and are designed for people who are in such poor health that they would receive little benefit from CPR.

But even with a living will and a heart-to-heart talk about what your loved one wants, given a life-ending diagnosis, it's still unchartered territory. None of us really knows until we're going through it.

So to help guide you, let's review what researchers found when they actually talked to people who were dying and asked them what mattered most.

What Dying People Want

In a compassionate and comprehensive study by the Veterans Affairs Medical Center in Durham, North Carolina, researchers interviewed dying patients and their doctors, social workers, hospice volunteers, chaplains, and family members. They asked what makes for a positive end-of-life experience. This is what they learned:

"I want to live without pain." Fear of pain was actually greater than fear of dying for many patients. As a result, preventing pain took center stage in their quest for positive end-of-life care. However, patients did not want pain medication that would send them off into a drug-induced haze. They sought to be comfortable so they could enjoy the moment and be able to fully experience the time they had left with their loved ones. Doctors and nurses were key to helping them manage their pain, and they appreciated those who reassured them that their pain would be controlled anytime, anywhere. They especially feared being without pain medications and treatment in the middle of the night.

"I want to make decisions about my care." The last thing dying people want is for family members to talk about them as if they are not in the room. Nor do they want to be spared the truth. Patients want to be involved in making decisions regarding their treatment. Gone are the hush-hush days of "saving" the patient from the diagnosis, tests results, and the subsequent prognosis. Supporting patients who are able to make decisions and take charge of their care relieves families of guilt if the patient desires less treatment and prevents conflicts and debates among family members who may not be ready to let go. Instead, what the patient wants becomes the unifying rallying point.

Tip You can't make good decisions unless you are well informed. Sometimes that means asking some tough questions. If a treatment is offered, ask about its goal. Will it gain more time, reduce pain, reduce the size of a tumor, or increase the likelihood of remission? That said, also ask about its side effects so that your parent can weigh the pros and cons and decide whether quality of time or quantity of time is more important.

"Tell me what to expect." Patients want to know the course of the disease and what to expect will happen to their bodies as the illness progresses. They feel that knowing is better than remaining in the dark because it saves them from being taken by surprise and frightened. They prefer to be prepared for what lay ahead than to be caught off-guard and having to make decisions in the midst of a crisis. Doctors and nurses who treated the patients also found that those who were better informed had a greater sense of control, which mattered a lot to them.

This also speaks to steps that you can take to better understand your parent's expectations. If it's been difficult for your mom or dad to bring this up, try this approach: "Mom, you know that I'm always hoping for the best, but let's talk for a moment as if your time is shorter than we planned. In that case, what would you want?" Then listen and don't rush in to fill the void if she doesn't speak right away. You might need to prompt her more by asking, "Is there something in particular you want to do? How can I help you do that?" You'll better understand her wishes, and she'll be able to remain in control.

"I need meaning in my life to make sense of my dying." Of course, this is a life-long search for all of us, but during end-of-life care, patients feel a deep urgency to express what life has meant for them. They seek solace from their faith, review their lives with family and friends by trading old stories and memories, repair relationships, spend time with family and friends, and say good-bye. If your parent is up for it and wants to meet with loved ones and friends, it would be helpful to make the arrangements sooner rather than later.

"See me as a whole person, not a diagnosis." No one wants to be seen simply as a disease, a diagnosis, or a case. But this is especially so when you feel that you are losing control of your body. A dear friend of mine who was seeing six different specialists during his end-of-life care—a nephrologist for kidney disease, an internist for his high blood pressure, a cardiologist for congestive heart failure, an oncologist for his cancer, and a wound doctor for a sore that wouldn't heal—said he felt like a bag of body parts. No one really saw him as a whole person, and his family was becoming worn down from all the office visits.

"I need to help my loved ones." Patients also reported that it was vital for them to contribute to the well-being of their loved ones. They found it comforting to be able to help them come to terms with their dying and accept the inevitable. And it was tremendously satisfying to know that they were able to leave behind the means to meet their family's physical and financial needs. They needed to know that the people they cherished most would make it without them.

MISC.

Legal Guide for the Seriously Ill: Seven Key Steps to Get Your Affairs in Order

The National Hospice and Palliative Care Organization with the American Bar Association wrote this practical, easy how-to guide that navigates families through the essential steps of getting their affairs in order. The seven steps show you how to pay for your health care, manage your health and personal decisions, administer your money and property, plan for the care of dependents, know your rights as an employee and patient, and complete various legal documents. Copies are available only online; you can download or read it on my website at www.lindarhodescaregiving. com under "Caregiver Tips."

Overall, patients want to be treated honestly by being given accurate information, no matter how difficult its message. They and their family members can make plans based on that information—taking a last vacation, deciding whether children take a leave of absence from school or jobs, or determining whether to pursue life-extending treatment. If the information is sugarcoated or overly optimistic, dying patients might mistakenly conclude that they have more time, resulting in treasured moments and future memories being missed. The more common regret among physicians and nurses is watching patients struggle with pain.

The Painless Promise of Palliative Care

As you've already learned, managing pain is a primary concern of every person facing a life-ending diagnosis. So it is with their loved ones; no one wants to helplessly watch Mom or Dad suffer.

Palliative (pronounced *pal-lee-uh-tiv*) care focuses on relieving pain, symptoms, and stresses caused by a serious illness, to give patients the best quality of life possible. For patients facing cancer, the oncologist will likely call in a pain-management team that includes physicians, pharmacists, and nurses. The team's goal is to find the most appropriate combination of medications to help your parent remain as comfortable as possible. They are experts at knowing how certain medications interact with each other and how they respond in conjunction with treatments like chemotherapy or radiation.

> **Tip**
>
> Who is the point of command? If your parent is seeing a number of specialists while receiving end-of-life care, it's vital that one physician act as the central point of command. Ask the primary care physician who should play that role. Questions to ask include: Who do I call when I think there's a problem and I need fast answers? Who receives all the results of the tests, lab work, and treatments, and interprets them for me? Who informs the other doctors of the status of my parent's condition and treatment? Who's responsible for coordinating the care?

Managing pain isn't just up to the professionals; it also involves your parent and coaching from you. The palliative care team must also rely on your dad's personal assessment and description of his pain. Not until they understand the nature and degree of your father's pain can they diagnose and prescribe the most optimal treatment plan for him. The team might ask him to keep a pain diary. Here are some of the things he should keep track of:

- The time of day he felt the pain. Does the pain change during the day or night?

- Did he experience any symptoms before the pain (for example, flushing, dizziness, or nausea)?

- Was he doing anything before the pain (for example, eating or getting out of a chair)?

- Where was the location of the pain?

- What ranking was the pain, on a scale of 1 to 10, with 10 being the worst? (He should ask his doctor for a pain rating scale so they are both on the same page.)

- How quickly did the pain come, and how long did it last?

- Did anything reduce the pain (for example, ice, heat, massage, or medication), and how much did it reduce his pain (using the rating scale)?

- How long did any of the pain relief measures relieve his pain?

- What did the pain feel like (for example, stabbing, burning, electric, throbbing, dull, or aching)?

With this type of diary, the pain-management team can identify patterns and find the root causes of the pain. The diary is also a way for your father to take some control over his illness.

Palliative care teams frequently tell their cancer patients to report their pain early and not wait until they can't bear it any longer. If you wait that long, it is more difficult to get ahead of the pain and reach a plateau of comfort. Let your parent know that this is one time he or she doesn't have to "buck up" and tolerate the pain.

Besides pain medications by mouth, the palliative care team might decide that the best way to treat your loved one's pain is to prescribe a patient-controlled analgesia (PCA) pump that continuously dispenses small doses of pain medication intravenously. If your parent feels pain that breaks through despite receiving continuous medication, he or she can simply push a button to receive an extra boost of the painkiller. If the pain is severe, the pain team might recommend that the pain medication be delivered directly into the spine (intraspinal) through a pump that is placed either under her skin or internally.

When to Call in Hospice

I've had patients and family members tell me that even though they know that *hospice* care is a good thing to do, they hold off because they think that it signals to their loved one that they've given up all hope. Neither the person dying nor the family members want to let the other down, so they keep up a front and hold off calling for hospice care.

Hospice brings together medical care and combines pain management and emotional and spiritual support for terminal patients with a life-ending illness and their families. This care is provided in the patient's home, when possible, or in an inpatient hospice facility with a homelike setting. The mission of hospice staff and volunteers is to address a patient's symptoms with the intent to promote comfort and dignity. They are experts at pain management.

But it really isn't about giving up hope. It's about working with a compassionate team that can manage pain, coordinate care, and address all those "what dying people want" hopes and wishes that we talked about earlier.

Today oncologists and family physicians are much more open about telling patients the status of their disease, including how much time they might have left.

If your mother, for example, views hospice as a way to reduce your dad's unrelenting pain, and if your dad sees it as helping your mom coordinate all his care, they each might see hospice in a new light. You can also reassure your mom that if your father decides to pursue treatment to extend his life (for example, with chemotherapy or radiation), he can opt out of hospice and return later.

There's another advantage to hospice care: Medicare will also cover respite care for your mother as long as your dad is receiving hospice care. Thus, if your dad needs to stay in a skilled nursing facility, in-patient hospice center, or hospital to provide him palliative care in order for your mother to get a break, Medicare will pay 95 percent of the Medicare-approved amount for inpatient respite care for up to five days.

Beyond the physical care provided, hospice volunteers and staff can help you understand what your loved one is facing and how he or she is coping. They can also help you and other family members handle your own emotions. Many of us are at a loss regarding what we should do before and at the time of death. The guiding hand of hospice nurses can help you through it at your own pace. They also stay in touch with you following your loved one's death and offer support groups during the process.

Medicare does provide a hospice benefit that covers almost all the costs of caring for a dying person during his or her last six months of life. To qualify for the Medicare hospice benefit, the following criteria must be met:

- Your parent must have Medicare Part A.

- Your parent's doctor and the medical director of the hospice must confirm that your parent has a life expectancy of less than six months.

- Your parent must agree in writing that he or she will not pursue any treatments to cure his or her illness.

The Medicare hospice benefit covers skilled nursing services, physician visits, skilled therapy (for example, physical, speech, or occupational), medical social services, nutrition counseling, bereavement counseling, 95 percent of the cost of prescription drugs for symptom control and pain relief, short-term inpatient respite care to relieve family members from caregiving, and home care. Medicare does not cover 24-hour 'round-the-clock care in the home; however, in a medical crisis, continuous nursing and short-term inpatient services are available.

Your parent's physician should be able to refer you to a good hospice. You can also visit the National Hospice Organization website at www.nhpco.org and click a map that identifies the Medicare-certified hospices in your area. You can also call Medicare directly, at 1-800-633-4227, or look in the Yellow Pages under "Hospices."

Here's a list of questions to ask:

- Are you Medicare certified? (If not, Medicare will not pay.)

- Are you a member of any professional organizations, or are you accredited?

- Do patients and families have to meet certain conditions to enter the hospice program?

- Are you willing to come to the home and conduct an assessment to help us understand whether this is the best option for my parent?

- What specialized services do you offer, such as rehab therapists, family counselors, pharmacists, and used equipment?

- What are your policies regarding inpatient care? With which hospital(s) do you have a contractual relationship, in the event my parent would need to go to the hospital?

- Do you require a primary family caregiver as a condition of admission?

- What are the caregiver's responsibilities as related to the hospice?

- What kind of emergency coverage do you offer? Who is on call? Will a nurse come quickly to the home, if needed?

- What out-of-pocket expenses can we expect?

- Will your staff handle all the paperwork and billing?

- What are your policies on the use of antibiotics, ventilators, dialysis, and/or nutrients given intravenously?

- What treatments are outside your hospice's purview?

Take the time to visit with the staff and tour the inpatient facility. The journey you are about to take will leave you with a lifetime of memories. Make sure you feel comfortable and at peace with the hospice professionals who will guide you.

Essential Takeaways

- Most people go through five stages of emotions when faced with a life-ending illness, known as DABDA by Dr. Elizabeth Kübler-Ross: denial, anger, bargaining, depression, and acceptance.

- What matters most to a dying person is controlling the pain, retaining the ability to make decisions, being told what to expect, being seen as a whole person, and helping assist loved ones in coming to terms with the person's death and making arrangements for their welfare.

- Hospice care can perform three vital functions during end-of-life care: control pain, manage and coordinate care, and help families through the emotional terrain.
- Medicare covers almost all the costs of caring for a dying person who is facing a life expectancy of six months or less. Accepting a hospice benefit means that the patient will not pursue life-extending care such as chemotherapy or radiation.

PART 4

Family Dynamics in the Swirl of Caregiving

Caregiving is a family venture. Often we don't realize how much of a generational gap we have with our parents. Nor do we appreciate how much coming of age during our own generation influences the views we have and the choices we make. The same holds true for our parents. It can explain why you may experience a tug-of-war between independence versus safety, privacy versus hired help, and a host of other elder care conflicts.

Caregiving issues have a way of calling up emotions that lay dormant for decades, and they often involve your siblings. Old rivalries, the sting of hurtful words, and personalities that just rub each other the wrong way can challenge the best of families to work in tandem while caring for aging parents. Add to this adult children living long distances from Mom or Dad, juggling careers and families, and negotiating with blended family members, and you get some interesting dynamics.

In Part 4, you get a heads-up on your parent's generational influences and learn how to side-step the common missteps between baby boomers and the Greatest Generation. Gain a better understanding of your relationship with your siblings, refocus your childhood, and find ways to work together. Finally, learn how to set realistic expectations and explore options when it comes to balancing your work life with caring for your parent and all the other older relatives in your family.

chapter 13

Working Through the Generational Gap

You and your parent's generational identity

How baby boomer values influence caregiving

How the Greatest Generation perceives caregiving

Bridging the generational divide

When it comes to family, we easily recognize the age differences: the kid sister, the older brother, aunts and uncles of all ages, the grandparents, and, in more families today, great- and great-great-grandparents. But often we don't make the connection to how much growing up in a specific generation affects our daily decisions and how we interact with each other.

Caregiving brings together multiple generations. The two that interact most closely are baby boomers and their parents, most of whom are members of the Greatest Generation, also referred to as the World War II Generation and the Silent Generation. Gaining a better understanding of how our generational experiences influence the way we relate to each other during one of the most challenging family undertakings of all will yield more compassion, patience, and appreciation. And who couldn't use some of that?

Describing the Generations

Generations are made up of population segments that generally span a 22-year period. Basically, that's enough time for one generation to begin replenishing itself. Growing up and going through life amid that age group has a profound effect on our personalities. Some demographers think it has an even greater impact than gender, race, or region. Why? Because world events shape our worldview, especially when they occur during "coming of age" years when we're in our preteen and teen years.

Older people fall into one of two generations these days: the G.I. Generation, or what Tom Brokaw coined "the Greatest Generation," born between 1909 and 1928; and "the Silent Generation," born between 1929 and 1945. Both age groups faced the Great Depression and its aftermath. They went to war or, on the home front, went to work; huge numbers were women who changed the course of family life. The G.I. Generation returned from the war to raise families, locating them to a novel kind of community, the suburbs, and gave them brand-new homes. They went on to discover vaccines for polio, tuberculosis, and whooping cough. They proudly held blue-collar jobs and led the movement toward worker's rights and unions. Many held the same job for their complete working life. Their diligent, hard-working, "get it done" ethos fostered one of the most economic booms of all times.

MISC.

Generational Identity

"No matter how contrasts between generations have been created, one fundamental fact of life remains true in the United States: Generations matter. To understand other people, and even to fully understand ourselves, we must consider generational identity at least as carefully as we consider any other social characteristic. And a salient part of generational differences in identity may be captured by contrasting generations' demographic experiences."

—Elwood Carlson, "20th-Century U.S. Generations," United States Population Reference Bureau, 2009

Those life experiences fostered a set of values among these two generations that you undoubtedly see in your interaction with your parents and grandparents.

Values of the Greatest Generation include the following:

- Respects and accepts authority
- Believes in rules and logic
- Lives by a defined sense of right and wrong
- Venerates discipline and hard work
- Prefers hierarchy
- Takes pride in self-reliance
- Saves money and values passing on an inheritance
- Admires loyalty to God and country
- Frowns upon complaining or bragging
- Values privacy; won't express inner thoughts
- Finds comfort in formality

When it comes to caregiving, we explore later how these values play out between the Greatest Generation and baby boomers. But first, let's take a look at the life experiences that framed the values of the largest generation of the century.

Baby boomers (born from 1946 through 1964) grew up with the *Mickey Mouse Club, Ozzie and Harriet,* and *Father Knows Best,* but their teen years turned radically different dancing to *American Bandstand, Soul Train,* Elvis, and the Beatles. Whereas their parents valued discipline and hierarchy in taking up arms against Hitler, baby boomers raised fists against their own war and took to the streets in protest. Hippies, long hair, psychedelic drugs, rebellious songs, and feminism dominated the culture.

They saw their parents' generation land on the moon and believed that they, too, could reach for the stars. And their parents made it possible by sending them to college in droves, both young men and women. But they also grew up with fear, ducking under desks during Air Raid drills to protect themselves from the ever-anticipated Russian atomic bomb that was nearly realized during the Cuban Missile Crisis.

The you-can-do-anything mantra of their generation was shaken with the Kennedy assassination and nightly televised death counts of Vietnam veterans. It became a generation that learned to live in the moment and "love the one you're with." Baby boomers became a diverse group and went on to engage in some of the most dramatic social change in any generation's history: the Civil Rights Movement, Peace Movement, and Women's Movement.

Values of the baby boomer generation include the following:

- Believes in individual choice and freedom
- Favors collaborative decision making
- Strives for self-actualization and improvement
- Prefers consultation over authority
- Respects flexibility and adaptability
- Seeks social involvement and inclusion
- Organizes work and life around goals
- Motivated to succeed; works hard to climb the career ladder
- Views life positively
- Fights for causes and is civically engaged

Baby boomers enjoyed adulthood in relative peace and did not face a global war as their parents did. Add to this their exposure to mass media, education, technological innovations, and world travel, and it's no wonder they've garnered a worldview unlike that of any other generation. It also influences how they see aging for themselves and how they tackle it for their parents.

Now that we know some of those defining demographic experiences that each generation faced and the values that ensued, let's take a look at how they influence both generations' mindset in giving care and receiving it.

Baby Boomer Missteps

Not long ago, I spent three weeks with my mother at a rehabilitation center in Phoenix. As she recovered from a broken leg and shoulder from two separate falls, other women were recovering from broken bones from osteoporosis. We'd have our daily lunch with her new "girlfriends," and their conversations became quite the eye-opener for me. Each of them had daughters and sons, all of whom lived out of town and, like me, had careers and families. Some would fly in to visit or were busy making plans for when their mother would go home.

But the stays were short and harried as they juggled jobs, husbands, and kids. The mothers were appreciative, but they also expressed resentment because these sons and daughters, though well intentioned, were being, in their minds, too bossy and too quick to make decisions; the children didn't trust the doctors, didn't listen to their opinions, and simply intervened too much. When they explained what their sons or daughters were doing, I quietly thought to myself, "Sure makes sense to me," and I imagined how it was playing out in their heads: "Why won't my mom listen? Why is she so stubborn? Why doesn't she appreciate all that I'm doing?"

The more I came to know these women, listen to their stories, and witness their fierce struggle to gain back their independence and free themselves from walkers and wheelchairs, I learned that there really is a generational gap in how we communicate about and tackle caregiving. Most of us start with good intentions; we love our parents and want to do well by them, and they want to do well by us. But if we really don't understand each other, it won't take long under the duress of illness, frailty, and caregiving for misunderstandings to make those good intentions all for naught.

So what baby boomer misconceptions get in the way of communicating with our parents? Let's link back to the values of the Greatest Generation and decipher how good intentions become misconstrued between the two.

See a Problem, Fix a Problem … Quickly

Your parent just fell and broke a hip, and once she comes home from rehab, you feel that she shouldn't live alone any longer. You look for assisted living facilities and bring her brochures from all the places you visited. You researched each one, and they met all the quality markers: she can make new friends, she can afford it, and she'll be safer. But she doesn't want any part of it. Or you swoop in on a visit and see that the old carpet is frayed and she has her furniture positioned in ways that will cause a fall, so you start rearranging things. And again, she won't have any part of it. Her appetite is poor and she's not cooking, so you sign her up for Meals on Wheels, but she promptly turns them away.

Baby boomers are problem solvers; they multitask, and they are known workaholics. Even though they participate in teams on the job and value collaboration, when it comes to their parents, somehow all that teamwork goes out the door. Part of it is in response to seeing their parents as frail and in need of help, so they quickly go about fixing their problems. As a result, sometimes they overreact and try to solve a problem that could work itself out or might not need fixing at all. They could also do too much and send their parent down a path toward dependency. Or they risk infantilizing their parent, which is never a good thing. You are never your parent's parent.

Quick fixes are also influenced by baby boomers' very busy lives; they don't have time (or so they think) to sit down and go over a list of options with their parents, wait for them to digest the pros and cons, and then make a decision.

They take matters into their own hands and just get it done, only for their parents to undo it. If they act too quickly, they might come up with the wrong solution: Mom might be acting confused not because she has Alzheimer's, but because the new pill she's taking is causing it. Subsequently, the fire drill to find a nursing home was unwarranted.

MISC.

Juggling Jobs and Caregiving

According to the Family Caregiver Alliance, the average caregiver spends 20.4 hours per week providing care. Among those who work, 70 percent have had to rearrange their work schedules, and 1 in 10 have had to reduce their work hours or take a less demanding job. Because of the economic downturn of 2008, 60 percent of working caregivers are now less comfortable taking time off work to care for loved ones, for fear of losing their jobs.

Because boomers value adaptability and flexibility, they don't understand why Mom and Dad can't make a few changes that are really in their best interest. And given their proclivity toward social inclusion, they don't see why their parent wants to remain at home, isolated and alone.

Question the Doctors, Search for Experts

Every time my 91-year-old father brings me along to a doctor's appointment, he begins with a disclaimer: "Linda's the boss—I just let her handle things." He says this because he doesn't want the doctor to blame him or think he's being impolite when I start asking questions. He dreads the possibility that I will suggest getting a second opinion because he believes that will insult the doctor who will never talk to him again.

Remember, this is a generation that doesn't question authority and likes knowing that someone is in charge. They respect and thrive in a world with rules and order. "Tell me, Doctor, what's wrong and how you'll fix it" works just fine for them. They aren't interested in searching for different hospitals, tracking down clinical trials, or traveling to specialty clinics—unless the doctor says so.

But baby boomers view doctors in a consultative role and explore their options—not just with one doctor, but with one or two others. They'll ask their friends and colleagues at work for referrals, and they'll jump on the internet to conduct their own research. They'll show up at appointments with a slew of questions, and some make their doctors cringe with copies of treatment recommendations they've found on the web.

All this "due diligence," from boomers' perspectives, makes their parents' generation downright anxious and frightened, because there is no social order in it. It's one reason parents hold back giving information to their overly diligent boomers.

No Reaction Means They're Okay with It

The Greatest Generation frowns upon complaining. They see it as whining and weak. Boomers see it as speaking up, or commiserating with friends to show they can feel each other's pain. Even when the G.I. Generation goes to a doctor's appointment where they're supposed to "complain," many downplay their symptoms or just chalk it all up to old age. This is why young geriatricians are trained to ask explicit questions to draw out what an older patient really feels. Men, especially, think they should just "tough it out"; as a result, a serious, deadly symptom might go unchecked.

Your parents might do the same with you, but for other reasons. They might want you to believe that they feel fine because they fear you'll force them to make decisions they don't want to confront, such as where they live, what they eat, or which doctor to see. Or they might simply not want to bother you because you have so many obligations yourself. The last thing they want to be seen as is a burden. So the Silent Generation stays silent.

Let's Hire Some Help

One of the most frustrating clashes between these two generations arises over hiring help. Whether it's simply to do household chores that are no longer safe to perform, to provide much needed personal care to assist with the tasks of daily living, or even to provide essential nursing care, the values of self-reliance and frugality halt many a baby boomer's quest to hire help. The parents who have managed to do things without relying on anyone to assist can't justify paying someone else to do something that they feel perfectly capable of doing. Of course, that's the rub: they might no longer be capable and are placing themselves at risk.

Boomers who do spend money on self-help items, such as cleaning, laundry, and services to make their lives easier and convenient find it hard to relate to parents who won't spend the money, especially when they can afford it. In fact, they come to resent their parents' asking them to do the tasks that boomers think they should be paying to have done. The parents consider it the family's job, not a task to hire strangers to do.

Remember, too, that this generation also values privacy, so they'll hesitate to bring strangers into the home.

Perhaps you can now see how generational differences create missteps by baby boomers on their caregiving venture with their parents.

Greatest Generation Missteps

The Greatest Generation also has its own missteps based on their generational values that cause tension with their well-meaning boomer children. Let's explore them.

Disregard Risks

One of my saddest moments when caring for my mother at the rehab center was when she asked the physical therapist, "Will I ever walk again?" My mother had broken her leg and had severe neuropathy and osteoporosis. In four months, she had broken four different bones, each from a separate fall. It wasn't his answer that was sad—in fact, he was hopeful. It was what she said following her question: "Linda's given up; she wants me to stay in this wheelchair."

My heart sank. I wanted my mom to dance again, not just walk. But she had fallen 10 times over the past year, and each had resulted in an injury. With neuropathy, her legs could give out without any warning; not even a walker or a quad cane could protect her. Yes, I wanted my mom to use a wheelchair. To me, it was a friend, a cocoon, and a safe haven. Her neurologist had warned her that this day would come. I just didn't want to see my mother in more pain. And yet the woman who always gave me hope now saw her daughter giving her none.

Given her generation's fierce desire to remain independent and self-reliant (think John Wayne), it's not uncommon to hear baby boomers complain that their parents continue to place themselves at risk because they won't accept help, whether from them or from professional caregivers. Not until there's a crisis, like a hip fracture, heart attack, or stroke, will they let others intervene. But as soon as they recover, they resume the way things were and convince themselves that everything is just fine.

If a couple is involved and one of them is a primary caregiver, it becomes all the more difficult to change the dynamics. Now you must convince two people that there are risks, and the caregiver often begrudges anyone questioning his or her capacity. Authority and loyalty, values strongly held among this generation, can prevent them from seeing or weighing the risks that their independence yields.

More than half of all reported elder abuse and protective services cases in the United States are cited as "self-neglect" due to behaviors of an older person that threaten his or her health or safety. Cases commonly involve refusing or failing to provide themselves with adequate food, clothing, hygiene, medical treatment, or medications, and not taking safety precautions that place them at serious risk of harm.

Disregarding the dangers that a parent's lifestyle and negligent health-care choices can yield spurs another reaction that parents usually don't consider: resentment by their children for what they view are preventable and unnecessary consequences that can significantly disrupt their lives. I've listened to countless distraught daughters and sons complain in utter frustration that their parents continue to place themselves at risk. In one case, an elderly mother wouldn't allow a nurse to come once a week to organize her medications, so she overdosed, became dizzy, fell, and broke her hip. The daughter had to take vacation days off work and make arrangements to have her teenagers cared for while her husband was out of town on business; he even had to cut his trip short to return home. The cost of travel, the risk of placing her job in jeopardy, the anxiety of leaving her kids, and the added demand on her husband all seemed to be lost on her mother.

It's not that parents intentionally want to bring harm on themselves or want to disrupt their children's lives. It appears that the self-reliance of this generation has led them into unchartered territory with an aging body that's letting them down and a mind's eye that blinds them to the risks.

Ignore the Facts

Denial isn't always such a bad thing. In times of tragedy, it acts as a buffer while our mind sorts through the overwhelming reality that it must now confront—kind of like a "timeout." But denial can also wreak havoc.

Years ago, I helped design a breast cancer awareness campaign to convince older women to get mammograms. The core message of the campaign centered on a saying that older women in senior centers repeatedly told me: "What you don't know, won't kill you." It explained why they wouldn't get mammograms and so many other screening exams recommended for older people. Others would tell me, "Certain things are best left alone," as if they would be bringing cancer or some other dreaded diagnosis onto themselves if they went looking for it. It's no wonder that, despite the availability of mammograms through Medicare, hundreds of thousands of older women still pass up the opportunity to have their breasts checked.

Denial?

In a major study of 146,000 women on Medicare, just less than half of white women 65 years and older had at least one mammogram every two years. The numbers were even less among black, Asian, Hispanic, and Native American women. This is despite the fact that 75 percent of breast cancers occur in women older than 50 years and mammography is especially sensitive at detecting breast cancer in older women.

Besides denial, this older generation isn't facing the facts for other reasons. First, the facts can be daunting. No other generation has ever faced growing old at the degree to which this group has—it's no longer uncommon to live well into your 80s and 90s. We're seeing the human body break down in ways we've never witnessed. For a group of people who thrive on being resourceful and rely on order and logic, finding their bodies "falling apart" is an assault on their inner core of control. The fear of losing control lures them into ignoring the signs of aging.

Today's world of medical technology, specialties, test results, diagnoses, complex treatment options, and regimens can be intimidating to a generation that hasn't enjoyed the medical literacy of their children. Your parent might not be choosing to ignore the facts; he or she might simply not understand them. And given this generation's respect for authority, he or she won't ask for clarification.

Suppress Information

The high degree of value placed on maintaining privacy, not complaining, and remaining in control also leads this generation to withhold information from families and doctors. There are a number of reasons:

- They might have always been private people, handling their affairs on their own and going to doctor's appointments by themselves. It might not occur to them that they are becoming more vulnerable and should start including their spouse and other family members in their decisions and asking them to doctor's visits.

- They might want to protect their loved ones from "bad news." Chances are, they have been providers most of their lives and have been protecting their children from whatever they considered harmful to their welfare. They might think that their spouses just can't handle it, so they hold off telling them.

- They might not want to trouble their loved ones, especially busy baby boomers with children, spouses, and careers. The last thing the G.I. Generation wants is to be a burden on their loved ones—or anyone, for that matter.

- They might fear losing control, so they stay quiet to protect their position of power. Some believe that if they let their boomer children know their vulnerabilities, they'll swoop in and take over.

Use the "Parent Card"

This isn't generational; it's universal. Who among us hasn't used the "parent card" to get our kids to do something they'd rather not? In the circumstances surrounding caregiving, the "parent card" can take a number of forms. Mom and Dad might not appreciate the collateral damage that affects their baby boomer kids when they won't accept any professional help because they've grown up with extended families that were able to pitch in and rescue each other at a moment's notice. They think it's just natural to help your parents, and no one should have to pay for it.

Not all families are perfect, as we were led to believe with *Ozzie and Harriet*. Some families have lived with alcoholism, mental illness, physical abuse, and very poor parenting. Children grow up feeling guilty and ashamed, while the cycle continues to play throughout adulthood. In these instances, playing the "parent card" can be damaging. Parents might make children feel guilty or rely on guilt to motivate them to help in ways that are clearly against the children's interest. Or a parent might play up sibling rivalry or stoke the fires of old conflicts. These behaviors aren't unique to any generation.

And then there's the "parent card" that baby boomers play without their parents saying a word: "But look at what Mom and Dad did for me. I can never pay them back; it's the least I can do." In most instances, that's absolutely true—and it's why you're reading this book, why I wrote it, and why we'll take care of them, if they'll let us, until death do us part.

Finding Common Ground

Hopefully, gaining a clearer understanding of how your generational life experiences affect how you view and handle caring for your parents—and how they approach *their* aging—will bridge the generation divide.

Given each generation's values and characteristics, here are some tips to get in sync:

- Take the time to listen and observe. Read between the lines, because your parent might not be forthcoming with what's going on. You might need to ask something, but do so in a nonthreatening way.

- Before acting on any matter of importance, acknowledge your parent's position of authority and gain permission on what actions to pursue. Even a parent with mild dementia will welcome this level of respect.

- Find ways to reinforce your parent's sense of control. Let Mom or Dad know that you'd like to follow his or her wishes, even when he or she needs help. Ask your parent to share his or her wishes in such a situation. It will give you insights on what is important now and in the future.

- Ask if your parent would like you to look into medical conditions or research other topics that might help in preparation for doctor's appointments. If you accompany your parent to appointments, treat the doctor with the formality and respect with which your parent is accustomed.

- When it comes to hiring professional caregivers and people to perform chores or home health care, advocate for the same, consistent caregivers to see your parent. This generation values privacy and doesn't like strangers coming into the home. If possible, offer to be there when a helper comes for the first few visits. Let your parent know you're more than happy to be the broker with the agency, to make sure your parent has help that he or she likes and wants.

- Ask what your parent thinks before you act, and appreciate the fact that Mom or Dad is likely grappling with losses—loss of job, social status, the protector role in the family, privacy, and control of their own bodies. All of these are the bedrock of that generation's identity.

Essential Takeaways

- The most important lesson to learn from this chapter is to keep one thing in mind: it's not always personal—it may be generational.

- Before you begin to react to what you consider irrational or just plain stubborn behavior, remember that you're dealing with the "Greatest Generation" that honors independence and privacy.

- Don't be so quick to rush in and solve your parent's problems without listening to their concerns and being attentive to what they don't say.

- You may need to encourage your parent's physician to ask questions and probe further when it comes to asking your parent to describe their complaints.

chapter 14

Siblings and Caregiving: Making It Work

How birth order isn't what it's cracked up to be

Discovering that each of you has different parents

How caregiving with siblings comes with warning signs

Why working with siblings doesn't have
to be so stressful

Caregiving is rarely a solo act. Whether you want to or not, you will interact with your siblings. And if all the surveys on family caregiving hold true, one of the most stress-producing dynamics you'll encounter in caring for your parents will be in interacting with your siblings as you respond to your parent's caregiving needs. It doesn't always have to be that way, though. Throughout this chapter, we explore ways to keep your family intact and less stressed.

Childhood Revisited

None of us doubts that the way our childhood played out with our parents and siblings has had an impact on how we relate to other people, found our mate, made friends, and perhaps even chose our line of work. The debate is over how much of an impact it had.

Literally thousands of studies have examined the effect of birth order on personalities. Some scientists say it has a profound impact, and pop psychology conjures up tests guaranteed to predict your best love match based on birth order. Other behavioral scientists say that it's basically a bunch of hogwash. You're just as likely to understand your personality by reading astrological charts—it's the sign you're born under that matters, not your parent's roof.

Yet common sense and cultural views have formed widely held typecasts about what first, middle, last, and only children are like and how they evolve as adults. We use these "shortcuts" to explain each other's behavior: "He's the baby in the family—of course, he denies how bad off Mom really is."

So let's get these typecasts out on the table and have a frank discussion on what this really means for you and your siblings when it comes to taking care of Mom and Dad.

Does any of this sound familiar?

- **First borns.** Tend to be high achievers, leaders, motivated, and confident. Seek approval. Downside: Bossy and perfectionistic.

- **Middle borns.** Tend to be social, relate well to older and younger people, are successful in team sports, are somewhat rebellious, and thrive on friendships. Downside: Often feel left out in the family.

- **Last borns.** Tend to be friendly, understanding, fun-loving, and low-key; seek attention; and are laid back. Downside: Are often self-centered and too laid back.

- **Only born.** Tend to be a lot like first borns, but never have to contend with the give and take of siblings; are high achievers, diligent, and leaders; and have a low need for affiliation. Downside: Selfish and perfectionistic.

How should you take this review of birth order stereotypes? Certainly not literally—and maybe even with a grain of salt. Yes, you probably see some truth to the descriptions, but part of this is because we generate them and use them to explain why a sibling might act a certain way when you don't understand each other or you disagree. But using these shortcuts also shortchanges your sibling and your relationship with him or her.

One of the most respected social scientists on birth order, Dr. Frank J. Sulloway, wrote a seminal book on the subject, *Born to Rebel: Birth Order, Family Dynamics, and Creative Lives.* He explains that birth order involves so much more than just the sequence of when you were born within the family. It's influenced by gender, differences in age among your siblings, your brother or sister's size (for example, whether the kid brother was able to "beat up" his older brother), and the amount of resources your parents had to divvy up throughout your childhood.

Sulloway also found that "families exert their greatest influence by making children *different,* not similar" and that the layered experiences of birth order are really formed *outside* the family, not so much in it. What's the message? You might need to get reacquainted with your siblings. If you still see them through the lens of birth order when you were kids, you're working off an outdated script. How they applied their first or middle years to life *without* you or your parents has had more of an influence on who they are today than birth order itself.

Here are a few other factors Sulloway would have you consider when assessing your sibling relationship via birth order lore:

- If you come from a larger family, your parents had to share their time and resources among all of you. Chances are, the oldest and youngest got more of the attention. It wasn't a matter of playing favorites; it was about the amount of sheer time and energy they had to allocate.

- How your parents were faring financially during your childhood affected the kind and amount of resources they could bestow upon you. While your parents were young and making their way to support a family, they might not have as much to provide the first child—but 10 years later, the last child might have gotten bigger and better toys because Mom and Dad's paychecks were bigger and better. Again, the "playing favorites" card doesn't apply.

- Children adopt different roles in the family that are influenced by birth order, gender, and genetics. It allows siblings to diversify their skills and perform in ways that enable them to escape being compared to or competing against a brother or sister. Essentially, they find their own niche. For example, an older child might occupy the niche of being a surrogate parent taking care of younger siblings, or the youngest child might take on the task of feeding a pet and becomes the "pet lover" in the family.

- Children go through a process of deidentification, as a means of differentiating themselves from their siblings. So if the older two are good at a certain sport or are very conscientious in school, the third child might not choose any sport and might kick back on school work.

Escaping Parental Pressures

misc.

Some middle children report feeling less parental pressure and welcomed "flying under the radar" while their parents were cutting their teeth dealing with all the *firsts* of the eldest—first car, first curfew, first dates—and the demands of a crying baby cutting their teeth.

Because our society promotes stereotypes of birth order (and your parents might have bought into them), your parents might have had certain expectations of you that then became a self-fulfilling prophecy.

What's the bottom line? Birth order's influence on your personality and your relationships with your family members is much more complicated than how you fell in line in your parent's birthing sequence.

My hope is that, by gaining a fuller understanding of how your interaction with your sibling(s) during childhood was and was not affected by popular birth order beliefs, you'll see them in a more positive and realistic light when the going gets tough.

Mom and Dad's Role in Shaping Your Relationship

Relationships with brothers and sisters are incredibly layered. During the most formative years of our lives, we learn how to compete, love, fight, make up, tolerate, negotiate, play, laugh, tell on each other, and keep secrets from our siblings. How our parents guide those experiences and interpret, praise, and punish them adds even more layers. All the while, the core of genetics and predisposition to personality lay beneath, infusing whatever layers we add throughout life.

Let's take a brief look at how parents in a few key ways influence the relationship with siblings during their childhood. It might spark an insight and help you reassess how you interact with your brother or sister today. Once you've done that, you'll be better able to tackle the task at hand: taking care of Mom and Dad *together*.

Your parents are fallible, and they undoubtedly made some parenting mistakes, as do we all. An important step toward working with your sibling or repairing a long-fractured relationship is to recognize how Mom and Dad might have contributed to a strained relationship then and now. Let's review a few of the more common ways that can cause tension between and among siblings.

Gender Bias

During the era when our parents raised baby boomers, gender roles between boys and girls were quite defined. So beyond birth order, being a boy or a girl placed certain expectations and limitations on how you interacted in the family. It also set in motion how you relate to your siblings.

For example, my parents had the girls make the beds every morning, including our brother's. I was the oldest, my sister was in the middle, and our brothers ranked second and youngest. Birth order had nothing to do with parceling out this chore, as well as many others. It did, however, set in motion how we related to each other based on gender and became a source of friction while we were young. It took the feminist movement to convince my mom that the boys could make their own darn beds!

For the World War II generation, that kind of gender bias was typical. Think about it. Our dad sure wasn't in the delivery room coaching Mom to breathe after he graduated from Lamaze classes. Our parents also measured their success at being a good parent based on how well their sons fared in finding a career and their daughters did finding a well-employed husband. Of course, this is an oversimplified view, and the women's movement dramatically changed their daughters' opportunities and roles. But as our parents age and become more dependent, don't be surprised if they revert back to the roles they assigned to you as a child—even if you're the CEO of a Fortune 500 company.

What our parents' generation believed about gender roles plays out today in a classic complaint caregiver daughters make about their brothers: "Why is it that when my brother finally shows up to visit my mom, she livens up, acts better, and then goes on for weeks about how great it was that he came to see her. He stayed one day and didn't lift a finger!"

The story usually continues with the daughter lamenting that she's the primary caregiver, spending 20 hours a week in addition to her job caring for Mom.

So before you think that this is just more evidence that your mom is playing favorites with your brother, it might be due more to how she was raised and her views on gender.

Playing Favorites, Competition, and Labels

Most parents want to leave a legacy whereupon their children have become best friends. Nothing disheartens a parent more than seeing adult children fight and not speak to each other. But as the saying goes, "You can't pick your family, but you can pick your friends." In some cases, siblings would never pick each other as friends. They just don't get along—at best, they just get by tolerating each other at obligatory family functions.

But if you came from a family in which your parents clearly picked favorites or assigned labels to different children as "the pretty one," "the trouble-maker," "the smart one," and "the clown," it increases the likelihood that your relationship with your siblings will face tension.

If your parents openly fostered competition among you and compared you, as in, "Why can't you get good grades like your brother?" or "Why can't you be more like your older sister?" you surely have had to work through the aftermath of being pitted against each other as children.

As a child you might have been angry with your parents for doing this, but you were in no position to challenge them. However, you sure could displace that anger onto your brother or sister and not even know why. Worse yet, today you might feel the pangs of jealousy toward your siblings, the seeds of which were planted so very long ago.

So go ahead and think back to situations, gender roles, and messages your parents might or might not have intended that affect how you see your siblings today. Read over Chapter 13 for more clues to how your mom or dad influenced your relationship with your sibling. Imagine what your siblings' lives were like as children in your family. Were they teased or made to feel left out? How did Mom and Dad treat them? Remember, this exercise isn't about finding fault; it's about finding enlightenment.

Refocusing Your Sibling Lens

We arrive at adulthood when we see our parents as real people and learn to reconcile missteps they might have made in our upbringing. Instead of remaining angry or blaming them for our own relationship mistakes, as well-adjusted adults, we can assess those effects, separate from them, and take responsibility to develop healthier and more effective ways of relating. It's easier said than done and keeps many a psychotherapist in business.

MISC.

Caregiving's Transition

"The push-pull of this life passage, being pulled backward while pushing forward, can affect even the healthiest of us, but the more emotionally separate [from parents] we are, the easier it is to recover and return to adult relating."

—Francine Russo, author, *They're Your Parents, Too!*

When you're tossed into caregiving for an older parent or face a crisis in his or her care, it might be the first time you've interacted in a deep and meaningful way with your siblings since you left home. Out of the blue, you need to talk about serious matters and are expected to work together. Sure, you might have been seeing each other for family holidays once or twice a year, but small talk over Thanksgiving dinner doesn't lay the groundwork for making medical decisions, handling Mom's stroke, or managing Dad's dementia.

Whatever unresolved issues or hurt feelings you might have toward your siblings or parent, the stress brought on by caregiving can quickly land you right back at your childhood home some 50 years ago. An offhand remark by your father, or a guilt-tripping statement by your mom or your oldest sister discounting your insurance advice despite your expertise in the field, can reduce you to acting like a 10-year-old in a matter of minutes.

Our task for this segment is to see things in a new light when it comes to understanding and working with your siblings. Let's get started.

Recognize What You're All Going Through

You are watching your parents decline, become more dependent, and struggle with losses, and the people who raised you and coveted their independence now need *your* help. You might also face a major shift in roles if one of your parents can no longer fulfill the role of patriarch, buffer, or matriarch. This will cause a shift in family structure that we discuss in the next chapter. The shift is unsettling and can release long-held, bottled-up tensions among the entire family.

You're also facing your parent's mortality—maybe not imminently, but it's likely on your mind and your siblings'. Each of you will navigate this emotional terrain differently, as described in the stages of loss in Chapter 12. You'll need to be patient while some siblings catch up to whatever stage you've reached and appreciate their fear, pain, and emotional needs while they grasp the changes in their own personal relationship with *their* parent. This process will be different from yours.

 Tip
You might have the same parents and grown up in the same household, but each of you has a different relationship with your parents. Expecting your siblings to react and respond the same to the *parents you know* will likely lead to misunderstandings and heartache.

Whether it's with your siblings or your parents, one of the more helpful things you can do—for you and for them—is to take a step back and imagine their reality. What might be going on in their lives right now? What emotional triggers lie beneath their reactions? How must they be feeling? If you were in their shoes, how would you react? Where are they coming from?

By getting a glimpse of your siblings' reality and their perspective, you'll know how to better respond to their needs. You might also gain a greater understanding of what's really driving their behavior.

For example, your brother might be going through a rough patch with family finances, and you are upset with him that he's not helping out with your dad. For two weekends in a row, he hasn't come by to relieve you. He keeps making up lame excuses. He hasn't told anyone that he's now working two shifts to make enough money to pay for the mortgage. He actually feels ashamed. The last thing he wants his dad to know is that he's down on his luck.

Of course, you don't know this, but you might respond with a note of concern rather than anger: "Gee, Tom, it's unlike you not to see Dad and help out. Is everything okay?" You could also express your need without attacking him: "I'm really going to need a break next week—is that something you can do, or should I make other arrangements?" You could test the waters even further with "I guess something important must be going on— let me know if there's anything I can do." This tact gives your brother an opening to explain his situation because you aren't placing blame or guilt. Had you done this, he would have likely reacted defensively and perhaps attacked you (for example, "Last year I stayed with Dad a whole week, and where were you?"), neither of which would have met your or your dad's caregiving needs.

Or maybe your sister is dealing with a stressful marriage, and her husband has become resentful of all the time she has been spending away from him while taking care of your mother. You have a busy life, too, and because your sister has always handled the long-distance caregiving so well, you never even think to ask how it's going.

Before you react, take the time to be more reflective and delve further into where your sibling might be coming from.

Parents' Perceptions

If you think you have a clear view of how your parents relate to you and your siblings, or who your mother would choose to care for her among all of you, think again.

In studies by social scientists Karl Pillemer and Jill Suitor, mothers were asked to identify who among their children they would select to provide them care and why. Gender ruled the day. The mothers chose their daughters, and most explained it was because "that's what daughters do" and felt more comfortable with a daughter for care that was "intimate" and private, like going to the bathroom.

The mothers also said that feeling "close" to the child who would provide them care was important to them. By "close," they meant feeling comfortable in their interactions and sharing similar values and attitudes. When the researchers asked their adult children who they thought their mom would choose as their closest child, most of them got it wrong.

The moms also gravitated toward choosing a child who had already provided them care. No mother based her selection on past help that she gave a certain child and now felt it was time for that child to repay the debt. Adult children, however, did feel more obligated to square with Mom by offering to care for her.

This research and many other studies reinforce that the choices you and your parents make regarding who provides care, how much, and what kind is influenced by many factors: some emotional, some practical, some based on a World War II generational culture. It's rarely as simple as Mom or Dad playing favorites. So don't assume the worst before you react.

Refocusing How You See Your Siblings

Busy lives scattered across states or even across town can cause brothers and sisters to lose focus on each other's lives and relationships. When a health crisis hits and siblings regroup to make caregiving decisions on behalf of their parents, they might find that the person they thought their brother or sister was—isn't. It can be an unsettling experience or a pleasant surprise. But in either case, being aware and open will help you gain a clearer view than if you were to rely on an old and possibly scratched lens from childhood. Here are some tips on cleaning up that lens:

- Be aware of your emotional triggers when interacting with your siblings. If you're seeing red, step back and strip away those layers to assess what is making you upset.

- Zoom in on your siblings' current lives. Are they struggling with a job, family issues, a spouse, or children? What would it be like to walk in their shoes?

- Beware of the "I shouldn't have to ask" test. Parents use this yardstick to see whether you *really* love them. If you do, you'll read their minds, know what they need, and will dutifully do it. Siblings use the test to prove a point, or it's driven by pride: "Why should I even have to ask?" or "What? You're going to force me to beg for your help when you know full well what Mom needs?" Be up front and ask for what you need.

- People never respond positively to guilt. Sure, they might respond and appear to do what you want in the short run, but it leads to a passive-aggressive relationship, and that will backfire. Shaming your brother or sister into doing more or stepping up to act "right" is wasted energy.

- Refocus what you're asking for. If your brother has a bad relationship with your dad, don't ask him to perform one-on-one caregiving tasks for your father. Instead, ask him to help *you* so that you can provide care for your father. In this instance, make it about you and your relationship with your brother—not about what he should do for your dad.

- Accept fractured relationships between your parents and siblings. If you have a great relationship with your sister, but she and your mom fight and have never gotten along, don't try to repair it—you could lose on both scores. It's simply not your job to fix it.

- Sometimes you have to be the first one to make a move or leave an opening to change the dynamic with a sibling.

- Be realistic in your expectations. If you take the time to learn more about your siblings' lives and gain a greater appreciation of their relationship with your parent, you'll know what to expect from them rather than working off a make-believe family that just doesn't exist.

- If you're the primary caregiver and your siblings really don't get what you're living with, ask them whether they would spend three days providing care to give you a break. Even if you need to remain in the same city or they stay with you because the care level is too great for a hand-off, it will give them a realistic picture of your parent's caregiving needs.

A Realistic Mom

"My two daughters really never got along. It wasn't due to sibling rivalry; they just have extremely different personalities that rub each other the wrong way. A few years ago, I finally decided that it made no sense for me to insist on being together like some Norman Rockwell painting and have my daughters and their families come back home to celebrate the holidays. Rather than sharing gifts, we shared tension, anxiety, and barbs. So I decided to accept them for who they are. Now I have separate holidays with each of them, and it is so much more enjoyable—no more pressure to live up to a fantasy family or forced smiles."

Reacquainted and Working Together

Hopefully, by gaining more insight into your siblings' needs and their relationship with your parents, you'll be able to work together in providing them care. It won't always be smooth, but if you communicate fairly, honestly, and assertively (see Chapter 16), you'll have a reasonable chance of success. Providing care and making decisions together can also be an opportunity to become reacquainted, to see each other in a new light, and to reconcile.

When my youngest brother was told he had a Stage IV cancer out of the blue, our family came together in ways we had never done before. My parents had gone through a bitter divorce and had not spoken in 30 years. But through the earth-shattering realization that they were going to lose their "baby" and watch him leave two young children, they set aside their differences and reconciled. All of us—three siblings, our in-laws, and our parents—worked together to help my brother and his wife along a heart-wrenching 12-week journey that altered all our lives and ended his. We grew stronger as a family and learned how to settle old scores in the blink of an eye. At death's door, family feuds that loom so large have a way of being rendered petty indeed.

Many people report gaining a great deal of satisfaction and meaning from their caregiving. Yes, it can absolutely be stressful, but research and surveys also reveal that caregivers report feeing valued, needed, trusted, depended upon, appreciated, and respected. They also enjoy being seen as competent by those receiving their care and by health-care providers with whom they interact.

If you're the primary caregiver for your parent, hopefully you share similar experiences and feelings. Just be aware that one of the more common complaints that siblings who are not the primary caregiver make is that you don't allow them the opportunity to help. You'll complain about not getting enough assistance, but when they ask whether you need anything, you say everything is okay. Or you'll give off the vibe that everything is under control, so they assume they're not needed. It's a trap that many caregivers fall into because it seems like too much of a hassle to leave Mom or Dad in the hands of someone else. Parents receiving the care often feed into this cycle because they're comfortable with what's familiar and consistent—you.

But you do need respite, and if you have siblings who have offered to help, give them the opportunity to do so. There are plenty of tasks to go around, so review Chapters 3 and 4 to find ways to do so. If you're consistently excluding your siblings and there isn't a safety reason involved, take some time to reflect on what's motivating you in turning them down. Is something in your childhood still unresolved? What about a bit of jealousy or a chance to be seen as "the favorite one"?

Now a bit of advice for siblings who live long distances from a parent and have a sister or brother acting as the primary caregiver: Don't become what's known as a "rescue kid" or "fly-in." I heard this term used, and not so endearingly, by parents and health-care providers when I flew in to care for my mother. Lucky for me, my fly-in status was seen as a positive. But it turns sour when you try to "rescue" your parent from the health-care providers they see and trust or second-guess your sibling's caregiving.

When you visit your brother or sister who is providing the care for your parent, be reassuring and tactful in sharing any observations about your parent's care. Spend some time with both of them, ask to pitch in, and compliment your sister for all that she does. You could create an opportunity to learn more about her needs by saying something like, "Being here makes me realize how much you do and what your days are like. Some days must be tougher than others." Then let her talk and explore with her what makes the "tougher" days more difficult, to gain insights on ways to help her. You're also showing that you care by just listening and allowing her to vent.

A "Fly-In" Without Getting on the Plane

Here's an example of what not to do when you are a sibling that lives a long distance from your parent, based on a friend's experience:

"I couldn't believe my sister when she called my dad and me at the hospital when he was about to have an outpatient heart procedure done and told us to leave immediately. She'd found a 'better' hospital. She's a nurse living on the East Coast and had talked to a physician friend who, from 2,000 miles away, told her to see one of his colleagues rather than my dad's cardiologist. That may have been helpful three weeks ago, but at this point, all it did was upset my dad and raise his blood pressure. We got into a huge fight on the phone. My dad stayed put and successfully had the procedure."

The nurse daughter could have meant well, but it upset her brother and sister, who were on the ground overseeing their dad's care. Her last-minute "rescue" made them anxious and resentful.

Before you start spewing a list of how much Mom or Dad has changed, you could approach your sibling by gently asking for permission to share your observations: "While I'm here, is there anything you'd like me to look for as to how Dad's acting or feeling when I'm spending time with him?" You've placed yourself in a position of assisting your sister rather than second-guessing her or making her feel like she's missing symptoms that should be addressed.

If you'd rather just share an observation, begin with, "I noticed that Dad seems more confused in the mornings. I'm not here all the time like you—what's your take on this?" In this instance, you are identifying what you see, acknowledging her status as primary caregiver, and asking what she thinks. This approach is far more productive than "How come you didn't tell me Dad's so confused in the mornings? What's going on?" Now you're being accusatory and inferring that she's not on top of his care—same observation, but a very different approach. Guess which one will drag you both back to acting like kids again?

Here's advice I give. I call this the I-CLAN Strategy for relating to your siblings:

> **Inform.** Be informed and inform each other.
>
> **Compromise.** Problems have multiple solutions.
>
> **Listen.** Be alert to what your sibling is *really* saying.

Ask. Look for help by sharing caregiving opportunities.

Need. Be aware of each other's needs, to meet your parent's needs.

The following are caregiving tips for siblings:

- Always keep two principles in mind. First, focus on the task at hand—meeting your parent's needs. Second, you and your siblings each know a different parent.

- Use objective information and medical reports to discuss your parent's needs, such as the results of a geriatric assessment versus personal opinions. Addressing actual facts is less emotional and will yield more appropriate and accurate actions and responses.

- Everyone can contribute to the care of aging parents, near and far. The experience of working as a team on the smallest of matters might open the door to small reconciliations.

- Dividing up tasks, keeping track, and working on them together can reduce tension over the long haul. Take advantage of electronic personal health records, conference calling, Skype, and good old-fashioned phone calls to keep the momentum going and communication flowing.

- The sibling lens fogs up as soon as you stop talking to each other. It can lead to misunderstandings or allow parents to play siblings off each other to get more attention.

- If your parent has given you financial control (for example, power of attorney), provide regular and thorough financial reports to your siblings, even if they don't ask for it. Better to be upfront on how expenses are being handled for your parent than creating an environment of doubt and second-guessing.

- If your family is not able to communicate because fractured relationships prevent it, seek out someone to facilitate discussions between and among you. Even if you all express your opinions separately to the facilitator and do not interact with each other, you'll be much farther ahead. For strategies on finding a facilitator, see Chapter 6.

Sticking with the Plan

"Once everyone agrees with a solution, it should be written down and shared with everyone involved. I love my siblings dearly, but this experience of caring for our dad has taught me that I should never rob a bank with them because some of them (okay, *all* of them) have trouble sticking to the plan. They often do things that they think are helpful because of feelings of guilt or some other emotion, and so they deviate from what we all agreed to—and that inevitably causes problems with our original plan."

—One of four siblings caring for a father with early onset Alzheimer's

If your family has a good deal of dysfunction and the advice throughout this chapter doesn't seem to apply (for example, you have siblings with mental health, addiction, or disability issues that preclude their caregiving), reach out to friends and also seek professional help. It may seem simpler to you to just "gut it out" and do this on your own, but caregiving as a solo act is fraught with its own dysfunction and tremendous emotional and health risks. And if you are an only child, please take the same advice: Go find some worthy "siblings."

Essential Takeaways

- Don't always reach for the "default position" when it comes to deciding who does what caregiving tasks. Let go of birth order and childhood roles. Look for what skills you've each developed as adults, and then assign the tasks accordingly.
- Give emotional support to your sibling caregiver. Just the act of listening that allows them to freely vent can be a powerful show of support.
- Follow the I-CLAN strategy. Inform each other, listen, compromise, ask for help, and be aware of each other's needs, to meet your parent's needs.
- Friends can serve as family to help with caregiving, too.

chapter 15

Making the Family Dynamic Work

How blended families make for challenging dynamics

Discovering the ways of your stepfamily

Getting in touch with your caregiving style

Balancing work and family life: protecting your future

When an older family member is diagnosed with dementia, a stroke, heart disease, cancer, or any other debilitating illness, the entire family is affected. Whatever role that family member has played—whether as a leader, enabler, buffer, protector, nurturer, provider, spiritual guide, peacemaker, troublemaker, or teacher—a void is created.

In a quest to resume order, regain the status quo, and fill that void, some members assume one or some of the roles that the sidelined loved one normally performed. Others, likely a spouse or a daughter, help nurse the loved one back to health so he or she can resume fulfilling those roles. Everyone's goal is to restore family life as it used to be.

But what happens when that loved one never fully regains the capacity to fulfill his or her roles pivotal to a family's stability? When the caregiving needs cause ripple effects throughout the entire family system? Or when those ripples turn into shockwaves?

Many of you already know the answer because you're living through it. You change, and so does everyone and everything around you, even if just by a fraction. Some of the change can be managed, some of it causes growth, and some is actually harmful. Or, "It just is what it is."

Elder Care's Impact on Family Structure

Families today face role changes and caregiving demands never before imagined. Long life spans and women delaying childbirth have resulted in the so-called "sandwich generation" of baby boomers who can expect to spend as many years caring for an aging parent as they will raising their children. The problem is, they're doing both at the same time.

Women in their 60s and 70s who might have planned to retire are taking care of ailing spouses *and* parents in their 90s. Chronic conditions abound among the fastest-growing segment of the U.S. population—85-plus-year-olds, half of whom can expect a nursing home stay and a stint with dementia.

Against this backdrop of high demand and high need, the family structure has also changed, making caregiving even more complex. Since 1960, family size has become smaller as a result of baby boomers choosing to have half as many children as did their parents. Now there are fewer potential caregivers for the greatest age wave yet to come.

The Fallout from Divorce

Divorce rates have doubled between 1960 and 2000, resulting in four times as many more divorced women in their mid-60s and older. Being divorced often places these older women in economic jeopardy.

The spiraling divorce rate among all age groups has created family units that would be unrecognizable to our great-grandparents. A nuclear family of the early twentieth century consisted of two parents, their children, and possibly their grandparents. Today a family unit consists of mini-mergers that yield step-parents, stepchildren, half-siblings, stepsiblings, and additional sets of grandparents.

And remember all those growing numbers of divorced men and women in their 60s and older? Increasing numbers of them are remarrying late in life or cohabitating as "sweethearts," bringing together grown sets of families who also might have gone through a divorce and add another slew of stepsiblings for caregivers to commune or reckon with.

Dimensions of Blended Families

In some respects, all these newfound family members could make up for the depleting numbers of caregivers rendered by small family size. On the other hand, it can instantly double the number of those who need care within an already overly stretched family system. And who says that everyone will gladly respond to a call for "all hands on deck"? And would you want all those hands on deck when they've never worked together in the first place? We call these new kinds of families "blended" or "reconstituted"; you can read about my personal experience with having a blended family in the following story.

The phenomenon of how blended families confront caring for their aging parents became all too real for me this past year while, during a four-month period, I found myself caring for my divorced parents, who live 2,000 miles apart, and each of their "sweethearts," who faced their own health crises during the same time period. My parents—my dad at 91 years and my mom at 85 years—both found new partners late in life but chose not to marry. Because titles of "boyfriend" or "girlfriend" didn't seem to fit, they referred to their friends' status as "sweethearts." For the purposes of this story, I'll refer to them as Mary and John.

Each of my parents and his or her loved one have been living independent lives. I've come to know Mary and John very well and consider them part of our blended family. I've also gotten to know their children but mostly in passing and during family get-togethers. We don't see ourselves as stepsiblings because we had long been adults with families of our own when our parents found their new partners. Even if our parents had married, the stepsibling status wouldn't have had any meaning among our families.

continues

continued

While I was caring for my mom who had broken her shoulder, John was having heart problems. He wasn't very forthcoming about his symptoms with his family, but because I was staying with my mom and John, I witnessed his troubling symptoms and urged him to see his doctor and immediately tell his daughter. My mother was relieved that I was there to urge him to talk to his family, which simply wasn't how John normally behaved. I also didn't want to get caught up in knowing something was wrong and having his family ask why I had never contacted them.

On the other hand, I didn't want to go behind John's back and "tell on him." After several conversations, and using all the advice you'll find in Chapter 16, John called his daughter and subsequently had an emergency procedure to open a major blocked artery. For the first time, two of his children, my mother, and I were assembled as a reconstituted family in the waiting room while John had his procedure.

My mom and I respected his children's space and recognized that all decisions regarding his medical care belonged to them and their dad—no matter how much my mom and John had talked about what each wanted if things "went bad" beyond what their advance directives described. My mother found it rather difficult not to be seen in the role of "wife" when doctors chose to speak only to his children. However, John's son and daughter always explained to my mom what the doctors had relayed to them.

In the coming weeks, as my mother entered a rehabilitation facility to recover from her fractures (on the day of John's procedure, she fell and broke her tibia), and while John recovered while living with his daughter, I learned that I needed to be more sensitive to John's feelings about his role as caregiver to my mother. I discovered that his daughter and I would both benefit from working together to meet both of our parents' needs.

My caregiving partner has always been my sister; it never occurred to me to think of John's daughter as part of our team. Our lives—through our parents—are bound together, especially when a health crisis befalls either one of them. We really need to communicate more while things are going well so that we have a good foundation when emotions run high and decisions need to be made quickly.

Within weeks of leaving my mom, my father called because his "sweetheart," Mary, was not so well. She had been diagnosed with lymphoma and had moved in with my father during her treatments. The arrangement allowed her only daughter to continue working and not worry about her mom being alone. I had known Mary and her daughter for 30 years. But now my dad was worried and wanted me to help Mary and her daughter. The next day, Mary was admitted to the hospital and my dad, her daughter, and I found ourselves sitting in a waiting room outside an intensive care unit. I brought my father to the hospital following an endoscopy for his own health problems, and Mary's first concern when seeing him was news about his test.

For two days, we watched Mary rapidly deteriorate and I learned another dimension to my blended family. Because I lived out of town and had never saw the level of interaction my father had with Mary's daughter, who had lost her dad in her early 20s, I didn't know how close they had become. When the doctors came in to talk with her, she immediately wanted my father sitting next to her and held his hand while she heard the news. He held her when she sobbed, learning that her mother had just a matter of hours left. And this stoic, Irish Catholic man who taught me to "never let them know what you feel" had tears in his eyes as he connected with her heartbreaking pain of losing her mom. I never, ever had seen my dad cry.

In that instant, I realized my dad had another "daughter." She was an only child without a dad, and he had been looking out for her in his quiet way for years. It had completely escaped me. I had focused only on Mary and my relationship to her. At the funeral, my dad sat next to Mary's daughter and held her hand throughout the service while my siblings and I sat in another row behind them. Today she looks in on my dad, and I see her in an entirely different light. How could I have missed it?

I learned four valuable lessons while interacting with my parents' significant others:

- My parents are connected with their "sweethearts'" families in ways I am not. Their relationship can be deeply personal, and I need to respect and appreciate the dimensions of that relationship.

- Because our parents are older, their health crises and end-of-life care will bring our families and all their permeations together. It's in all our best interests to open the communication channels now rather than later.

- Families have their own culture and behaviors that are normal to them. Take the time to observe their ways and follow their lead when it involves their family member.

  John's family was more private and spoke to doctors separately. My mom, who is open and inclusive, had to step back and not take the exclusion personally. It was *their* way.

  Mary's daughter, who is an only child, wanted both my dad and me alongside her when she talked with the doctors. Once she heard the prognosis, she quickly reached her husband and children so that they could come to the hospital, along with her mother's brothers and their families, to say their last good-byes. Within an hour, 15 people became part of an open and supportive vigil. It was *their* way.

- You might have to step aside and keep your own emotions in check, just as if you are dealing with your own siblings. My confession? I felt a twinge of "sibling" rivalry when I went to sit down next to my dad, as I always do, at Christmas Eve dinner. He told me that this is where Mary's daughter would be sitting. Of course, she needed to be next to my dad—it would be her first Christmas without her mom, who had always joined us. What was I thinking?

When Blended Becomes a Battleground

Not all blended family stories end on a positive note as mine did, but it could have gotten messy if we had handled things differently. I've read countless entries on caregiving blogs and receive emails from my readers describing awful scenarios of fights among stepchildren and step-parents. For example, a stepfather has durable health-care power of attorney and places Mom in a nursing home even though her biological children completely disagree and want to take care of their mother at home. Or step-children argue over who should pay for what costs and, as a result, no one pays and Dad receives no care. Accusations fly among the clans over who is stealing what and from whom. No one agrees on who really has Mom's best interests at heart.

If your parent is about to remarry, make sure he or she has an advance directive, has a durable health-care power of attorney, and has had an open conversation with you regarding desired care and living arrangements if he or she suffers a stroke or is diagnosed with dementia or another illness that requires prolonged care. Use the "what if" scenario exercise (see Chapter 4) and commit your parent's wishes in writing.

If your parent is already remarried and you haven't had this conversation, have it now. The more openly you've discussed these matters, the less likely you'll encounter distrust, accusations, and resentment in the heat of making tough caregiving decisions. This kind of emotional drama shouldn't take center stage when your mom or dad's needs should be playing the lead role.

Caregiving Styles Within Families

Caring for family members who are ill and frail, whether young or old, certainly isn't a new phenomenon. It's ancient and part of humanity's code. But our attitudes toward caregiving and how we are able to perform it, given today's world of extended, blended, smaller, and long-distance families, has become much more complicated. This is especially so because many of our traditional caregivers, women, are working and raising children, too.

"Different strokes, for different folks" rings true when it comes to caregiving styles. Some people seem to come by it naturally; others have seen their grandmothers and mothers fill the role seamlessly and treat it as the natural order of family life. Most of us learn by trial and error. But no matter how we come by our style of caregiving, it has been influenced by our culture and the values our own families associate with being a caring person.

An insightful study by researcher and occupational therapist Mary A. Corcoran, PhD, appeared in *The Gerontologist*. It identified four caregiving styles by studying nearly 100 pairs of caregivers and their care receivers. Researchers interviewed the caregivers and studied their interactions by analyzing videotaped observations of them while providing care to their loved ones.

Sharing the four styles that emerged can help you identify which resonates the most with you and learn how different styles evoke different responses and results. Even though the majority (62 percent) of care receivers had a diagnosis of dementia, these caregiving styles are relevant to how many families provide caregiving in a broader context. Let's take a look.

Facilitating

You focus on the emotional health of your loved one, and if your mom or dad is the primary caregiver, you turn your attention to his or her well-being as well. You see your loved one as a productive and loving person who still has the ability to enjoy meaningful activities, and you promote this image of your loved one to others. You support your well parent's efforts to provide good care to your loved one, but you make sure he or she won't compromise his or her own health in the process of doing so.

A trademark of facilitators is their preference for involving their loved one in one-on-one activities such as enjoying a favorite hobby, cooking, playing cards, and gardening—anything that fosters cooperation and working together. Creating a comforting and secure environment is a top priority for you, and you facilitate it by using a calm voice, a warm sense of humor, and facial expressions that reassure your loved one that everything is okay. You consider providing information and caregiver tips that benefit your well parent's emotional health a vital role.

Overall, this style provides cooperative interaction, disseminates information that enhances the emotional health of caregivers, and cultivates an environment of reassurance to caregiver and care receiver alike.

Balancing

You see the whole picture and spend your efforts on balancing the needs between the care receiver and the caregiver. If you're the primary caregiver, you understand how important it is to take care of yourself as a means to take care of your loved one. You also see the caregiving ripple effects throughout your entire household and seek to keep the peace. You avoid sacrifice on the part of one person for the advantage of another.

In the balancing style, caregivers juggle a number of activities; for example, they work in another room while listening to the care receiver through a sound monitor, or they give their loved one an activity to do, such as a household chore, while they accomplish another task. Balancers are used to making trade-offs and sometimes feel conflicted while they manage multiple roles and schedules that demand their time and attention. They engage in activities that run parallel to their loved one's. It doesn't require the same level of interaction with the care receiver as does a facilitating style.

Advocating

You're vigilant about your loved one's well-being, and when you suspect a problem, you are right on it. You monitor your loved one's needs for help and respond in ways that assist yet still promote an appropriate level of independence. You observe your loved one's involvement in activities to assess his or her level of functioning and determine whether any action should be taken to address potential problems.

You advocate for your loved one by actively interacting with physicians, nurses, and any one else providing direct care. This style of caregiving is most often used when you're no longer providing daily one-on-one care. Many advocates whose loved one has transitioned to a facility devote their energies to "keeping an eye out" and "speaking up." But it's done in a way that's flexible and builds rapport with the staff so they'll look kindly on your loved one.

In an effort to garner respect for your loved one, you share old photos, accomplishments, and stories. You do this so the staff understands and appreciates your parent's history and, hence, gives him or her the respect and dignity deserved.

Directing

You focus on the physical health of your loved one overseeing nutrition, medical and medication routines, doctor's appointments, and hygiene, and making sure she or he receives the best medical care possible. You like to maintain order, so you set standards for what needs to be done and what health practices and behaviors your loved one should follow to stay healthy.

You're comfortable in giving directions and do so in writing or verbally. This style is different from a facilitator, who is more likely to provide directions by guiding and touching rather than by directing.

When you encourage social interaction for your loved one, it's based on what you perceive as beneficial for him or her and not necessarily for yourself.

Sometimes you feel frustrated with your loved one and your caregiving situation because it's difficult to maintain order or control declining mental and physical abilities. You remind yourself that this is the best you can do, given the circumstances.

No one, of course, follows a particular caregiving style all the time. You might use an advocating style when you're interacting with doctors; then by the end of the visit, you facilitate a discussion between your mom and dad to better understand what was said and grapple with the implications of a dementia diagnosis. Later that evening, you might balance your caregiving by asking your dad to bundle newspapers, which he enjoys doing, while you grade papers for the class you're teaching. You might need to direct him to take his medications and reassure your mother that she's doing all that she can. All in a day's work!

Different styles are appropriate for different circumstances, but it's likely that you'll gravitate to one more than another. Plenty of studies have shown that caregivers who take breaks and try to maintain balance in their lives tend to do better healthwise and emotionally.

Whatever style you use, make sure it has some component that includes taking care of yourself (see Chapter 5).

Working Families: Setting Realistic Expectations

One major cultural shift we haven't talked about is the impact that women in the workforce have on how families provide care. This matters because the majority of caregivers are women, many of whom are thrown into a juggling act that many simply can't withstand. Raising kids, sustaining a marriage, and maintaining a career is enough for anyone's plate, but add caring for one or two aging parents (which, on average, consumes about 20 hours a week), and you can expect the juggling act to end with a crash.

Men, too, are increasingly becoming caregivers, but the majority are in their mid-70s caring for an ailing spouse. Most baby boomers providing care to parents are working, and their employers report that their work productivity is lessened by nearly 20 percent; they also suffer from higher levels of stress, depression, and health problems than their colleagues who don't have parents needing care.

If you are a working caregiver, you might have had or are considering a number of alternatives to help you balance your family life with your job. Some of these might be the following:

- Let go of advancement or promotion opportunities.

- Reduce your hours to part time.

- Ask for or find a less demanding job.

- Pass up taking extra shifts to earn more money.

- Turn down new training opportunities that require traveling out of town.

- Expend all your personal leave, sick days, and vacation days to provide care.

- Take unpaid leave (Family Medical Leave Act).

- Resign from your job.

Because of the 2008 economic downturn, many workers are reluctant to take time off work to provide caregiving because they are afraid of losing their jobs or can't afford to lose the wages. On the flip side, some families are taking an extra job just to pay for the out-of-pocket costs associated with providing care.

In any event, before you take drastic steps, especially quitting a job, be aware that women who leave a job during their working years to provide full-time caregiving are 2.5 times more likely to live in poverty once they reach retirement age than women who remained in the workforce. These women can expect to lose an estimated $659,000 in wages, Social Security, and pension contributions, as well as lost coverage for health-care insurance over her lifetime (source: AARP Policy Institute).

My guess is that your parents certainly don't want this for your future, so consider taking these steps to achieve balance between your job and caregiving:

- Talk to your supervisor about your situation. If your employer has an employee assistance program, explore your options. Because of the huge numbers of workers faced with caregiving, companies are offering more assistance to their employees.

- Explore whether you can complete any of your work at home instead of at the office (telecommuting).

- Ask how you can use the Family Medical Leave Act (see Chapter 3) and how it can best complement the days you have accumulated for vacation and personal leave.

- Research opportunities at work, such as splitting your responsibilities with another co-worker (job sharing) in a similar situation or devising a more flexible schedule (flex time).

- Ask your human resources department whether it offers any information and referral services to help you track down benefits and resources to care for your aging parent. Human resources also might provide the services of a geriatric care manager (GCM) to help you create a caregiving plan.

- Look into the option of using an adult day center that offers therapeutic and social activities for your parent while you are at work.

- If you have siblings, create a Caregiving Resource Assessment Worksheet (see Chapter 3) showing how this impacts your job (for example, days you've been off work, lost vacation days, and so on). Discuss how they can help. For example, you all might contribute to covering a nonmedical senior care aide to assist or pay for adult day center services.

It's best to explore all your options at work before you walk away from your own economic security in your older years. Don't wait for your work performance to start slipping before you approach your supervisor.

New Times: Mom, Will You Hire Me?

Ever thought of being paid by your parents to care for them? Or pay another family member to do so? It might sound crass, greedy, and unloving, but as caregiving demands spiral out of control and a son or daughter loses a significant income to provide a parent care that allows him or her to remain in the home, it starts sounding like one of those win-win options.

Once parents realize the costs of assisted living or hiring someone to come in and care for them, they recognize that asking their son or daughter to give up their income so they don't have to spend money on their care isn't a fair trade. When adult children realize that they can prevent Mom from living in a facility she doesn't want by being compensated for their caregiving at a much lesser cost to her, they also feel better about exploring the option.

Some parents who have entered into *caregiver contracts* report feeling that they remain in control and no longer see themselves as a burden.

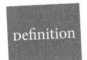

Caregiver contracts are legal documents between an elderly parent and a family member that spell out in specific details the kinds of services and tasks the caregiver will provide, over what course of time, and the rate of pay for the services performed by the caregiver.

If you choose this option, I highly recommend using an elder law attorney (see Chapter 8) to draft the contract. Make sure other family members are aware of what is being agreed upon. To prevent conflicts, this type of arrangement should be transparent to all the family stakeholders.

When drafting the contract, you'll need to address paying Social Security, Medicare, and unemployment taxes, which will include filing a W-2 form and determining terms of payment. The hourly rate should be comparable to what a private home care provider would charge in your area, which is usually in the range of $20 to $35. If your family member is a nurse or other medical professional, the rate can be higher yet, but it should reflect the level of services actually rendered. In other words, you can't charge $75 an hour because that's what you're paid as a nurse, when you're really doing household chores that commonly pay $20 per hour.

As a paid caregiver, you should keep a daily record of the tasks you perform and draft a report on your parent's status just as if you were working for a home care company. As an added protection for you and a benefit to your parent, pay a GCM once a month to review your care plan and daily reports to validate the performance of your caregiving. Also ask the manager to share professional advice on any changes he or she recommends for the care plan. Make the review part of your records, and share it with other family members.

Tip

To learn whether your state offers reimbursement for caregiving provided by family members, call the Eldercare Locator help line at 1-800-677-1116.

Some state public benefit programs now allow family caregivers to be compensated for providing care, and a growing number of long-term care insurance companies allow nonmedical senior care or nursing care to be provided by family members as well. So if your parent has such a policy, check whether that provision applies.

Essential Takeaways

- Living up to family images of a Norman Rockwell painting will bring you a great deal of frustration. Today's families are blended, extended, and stretched. Be realistic with each other.

- If you are part of a blended family, take the time to observe, appreciate, and respond to the ways of your stepfamily.

- Be conscious of your style of caregiving and how it affects the kind of care you provide.

- Before you make any major changes with your job, talk with your supervisor and human resources staff to explore a wide range of options to help you balance your work life with family caregiving.

Part 5

Communicating in Sync

You've known your family for a lifetime, yet when you're communicating with them, you may feel like none of you speaks the same language. However, if there's any time you really need to understand where each of you is coming from, whose best interest is being served, and how best to relate your thoughts and feelings, it's now.

Questions of whether Dad should keep driving, whether Mom should live alone, and why some siblings don't help are conflict-laden questions that a great number of families face. The caregiving choices that confront you, your parents, and other family members are also affected by money.

The greatest communication challenge any family faces is talking through dementia. Knowing what a loved one needs, interpreting what he or she means, and figuring out how to respond requires patience, understanding, and specific techniques that many caregivers must learn to develop. It may not come naturally.

In Part 5, you'll identify your communication style and learn what works (and what doesn't), pick up techniques on how to interact with a loved one diagnosed with Alzheimer's or another form of dementia, acquire a better understanding of the costs of elder care, and discover how your "money style" influences the choices you make and the disagreements you incur because of it. You will also uncover helpful strategies for talking through money issues that focus on the bottom line: Mom or Dad's best interest.

chapter 16

Reaching Accord: Styles of Communicating for Caregivers

Solid and sensitive communication skills needed in caregiving

Being accountable for how and what you say

Not owning other people's emotions

How assertiveness yields win-win results for you and your parents

Discussing caregiving and making decisions regarding options requires a great deal of communication. Whether it's talking to other family members or your parents, or conversing with physicians, home health aides, or a Medicare associate, being aware of how your communication style is received by others is good to know. This is especially true when it comes to working as a family to address the multiple caregiving challenges heading your way.

The Four Styles of Communicating

So what is a communication style? Several models describe four basic styles, each with its own interpretation on a common theme. The model I'm choosing to describe for you is more general and probably more familiar to you than those that management consultants use in work environments.

As you read through this review, make notes about what style seems to resonate the most with you. Be aware that you likely blend some of the characteristics of each style, given certain circumstances and social situations. Rarely does anyone neatly fit into just one style, and there are extremes to each. We choose styles depending on past experiences, how our parents communicated (or not), and which styles have met our needs and worked for us in our varying circumstances.

Your goal is to become more aware of how other family members will interpret your style when you're discussing caregiving issues. This will help you step back when emotions run high to ask yourself some questions: Is your style of communicating getting in the way? Is it adding fuel to the fire? Is it getting you where you want to be?

Passive Communicators

You care about other people's feelings and are a good listener. You're the one who usually appears calm in a crisis, with a quiet voice. You often place your needs last and rarely express how you feel or ask for what you really want. You hope that other people just pick up on your needs, and you may quietly feel hurt or resentful when they don't just "get it" and respond. You're an expert at hinting. You may think that your feelings don't matter, so why bring them up? In your mind, life is easier if you avoid confrontation at all costs, even if you're the one paying the price.

You're not expressing your needs, though, so over time, that can make you feel depressed and resigned to unsatisfactory situations. One day the cork might pop and you'll blow off steam that shocks your family members and you. If so, you'll soon feel guilty and be apologetic.

Because you're self-sacrificing and you rarely openly complain, people may read into this either weakness or kindness and come to you to do even more for them. You may interpret this as being needed and liked, which builds dependent relationships, or you could resent them for "walking all over you." You've learned that it's safer to stay quiet, to not express your feelings, and to hang in the background. Those strategies keep you unnoticed and in your comfort zone.

When it comes to facing a problem, you'll avoid it, deny it, downplay it, ignore it, or procrastinate so you don't have to deal with it. You do this not because you don't want the problem solved, but because it will likely involve different points of view and possible conflict that makes you anxious and feel like a deer caught in headlights. You'll sit on both sides of the fence for as long as you can.

Of course, this can make matters worse. When family members discover how bad things are, they may see you as ineffective, and you'll agree to allow them to take over. You won't speak up if they are handling things in ways you find troubling. In fact, you're used to displaying behavioral queues that make people think you're agreeing with them, while, in fact, you disagree on the inside. Underneath it all, you'll feel those familiar feelings of being hurt and resentful.

MISC.

Bumper Stickers on a Passive's Car

"Don't make waves."

"Don't rock the boat."

"Silence is golden."

When you do express your thoughts, you usually begin with, "I know this may sound stupid …" or "This is probably wrong, but …" and fully expect to be ignored. You'll tell yourself, "At least I tried," or you will simply slip into a self-fulfilling cycle of "No one listens to me, and I rarely get what I want." Taken to extremes, you will rarely offer solutions and may have trouble looking directly at another person; others might think you're either being shy or trying to hide something.

Aggressive Communicators

You confront difficult problems and don't hesitate to tackle conflict. You're known to be very persistent and are determined to win. You make it clear and in no uncertain terms what you want or think should be done. You really don't have much time for those who hesitate or don't just come out and say what's on their mind. But heaven help them if what's on *their* mind is contrary to what's on *yours*—you'll quickly show them how they're wrong.

When it comes to conflict, you take the floor quickly and dominate the discussion because you're always right—why waste the time looking for other solutions? As a result, listening is hard for you, and you tend to interrupt others, causing you to be seen as rude. Taken to an extreme, aggressive communicators quickly label people when they disagree and call them names, blame them, or criticize them for whatever they view as wrong.

Aggressive communicators aren't above humiliating people as a means of controlling them, and they spend a good deal of energy manipulating people to get what they want. In a family caregiving situation, you'll use the "guilt card" to draw people in or use it to push their buttons. In your world, using anger to intimidate is an effective way to get people to back down.

Bumper Stickers on an Aggressive's Car

"I make waves—enjoy the ride."

"It's hard being right all the time."

"It's my way or the highway."

When you express your thoughts, you usually begin with "You should …," "You'd better …," and "I know that …," and you fully expect to be followed. Instead of looking for solutions that are collaborative and win-win, you see everything from a win-lose proposition—and you aren't about to lose. Given your style, you'll likely be seen as bossy and a know-it-all, eventually losing relationships in your wake. This could result in family members not telling you the whole story so that they don't invite your ire or involve you at all.

Passive-Aggressive Communicators

As the name implies, you combine the characteristics of being both passive and aggressive. You gravitate to this style when you feel angry or frustrated, but you'd rather have everyone think that you're just fine. All too often, you say yes to a request when you really want to say no, and you resent going along. You don't want to confront the person or situation that's making you upset.

Rather than confront the person who is making you upset, you'll "get even" indirectly by finding ways to sabotage that person's efforts. You'll engage in gossip, make sarcastic remarks, or complain behind the person's back. You may have developed this style because you're uncomfortable expressing your feelings or because you've been shot down too many times and don't know any other way to stand up for yourself.

Bumper Stickers on a Passive-Aggressive's Car

"Whatever."

"Doublespeak is my first language."

"Revenge: the feel-good emotion."

You believe that you're defending your rights when you find ways to undercut someone who has offended you or bullied you into doing something you didn't want to do. A research study by Syneticsworld, an international management firm, found that if someone acts aggressively against another person, such as a person who ridicules them in front of others, within 20 seconds, the offended person will decide how to get even. Called the "20-second payback rule," it's a tactic you're adept at using.

When you express your thoughts, you may say things under your breath, be sarcastic, and use facial expressions that don't match how you feel, like smiling when you're really angry.

If you use this style, you'll eventually be "found out" and be seen as untrustworthy because no one knows what you really think or feel. And they'll fear you'll be manipulative with them, even if they're nice to you. Family and friends may complain that you play too many head games when it comes to relationships.

Assertive Communicators

You work hard to get people to work together and reach solutions that everyone will feel good about, even if some people must compromise. You care about relationships and invest heavily in them, yet you don't allow people to take advantage of you. You're able to say no without offending the person whose request you're declining. You're honest with your feelings and express them clearly, letting people know what you want and how you feel without demanding that you get your way. You listen because you inherently believe that you can work things out and that other people's views matter.

Whereas an aggressive communicator is all about expediency and "let's just get this done," you're in it for the long haul and consider how your actions affect the relationship or the situation. You can make requests for assistance from others without feeling guilty.

Because of your straightforward manner, people don't have to guess at what you want, and you're less likely to encounter misunderstandings.

MISC.

Bumper Stickers on an Assertive's Car

"There's no *I* in *Teamwork.*"

"Less *me* and more *we.*"

"It's not about getting credit—it's about getting it done."

When you express your thoughts, you usually begin with an "I-statement" that's told in a respectful way ("I feel that …"), or you'll ask for validation on what someone has just said ("Let me see if I understand you correctly …" or "Let's explore our options …").

Assertive communicators actively listen and engage in conversation, wanting to understand where the other person is coming from. You state observations instead of labeling people or making judgmental statements.

If you see a problem, you're proactive in getting those who have a stake in it to sit down and solve it. You have an open and natural demeanor, and people probably describe you as even-tempered and good-humored. Overall, you gain the most respect from being self-aware and honestly express your feelings so that people know where you stand without offending them. You also reduce the potential for misunderstandings because you are seen as authentic.

What's Your Style?

When you read over the four different styles, did you recognize yourself favoring one style over another? Is there one you seem to feel more comfortable using most of the time? When you're angry, which style do you use? When you feel hurt or unappreciated, which style do you use?

To get a better understanding of your communication style, recall an uncomfortable conversation that you've recently had with your parent regarding a caregiving issue, and answer the following questions:

- How long did it take you to have the conversation? Did you put it off?

- What was your greatest fear going into it? Did it happen?

- Did you feel better or worse at the end of it?

- How do you think your parent felt during the conversation? How do you think he or she feels now?

- Was the issue resolved?

- As you look back, was anything left unsaid? Do you know why?

- Would you do anything differently now that you're more aware of the communication style you used?

If you found yourself delaying the conversation because you were afraid your parent was going to get angry at you or that you might hurt his or her feelings, chances are you gravitate toward being passive. Did you avoid any further discussion when you felt that either of you was getting upset?

If you waited until your parent was doing something wrong so you could point it out to her and gain the upper hand, you're inclined to be an aggressive communicator. You probably have no idea how your parent felt during the conversation because, instead of listening, you were busy telling him or her what to do.

If you never really had a conversation, but instead dropped hints or made sarcastic remarks to get your parent's attention on what you really wanted to talk about, and then denied it and acted just fine, you used a passive-aggressive approach. The issue remains unsolved, and you're likely not feeling any better about it.

If you calmly asked your parent to sit down and talk with you, and shared how you felt about the matter that you wanted to raise in an open, give-and-take manner, you used an assertive style. Chances are, you really didn't fear having the discussion because you genuinely wanted to learn what your parent thinks. Both of you feel good about the outcome, and you know this because you've asked your parent.

Tip

If you'd like to take an online quiz to help you further analyze your communication style, go to my website (www.lindarhodescaregiving.com) and visit the resources section. You can also find links to videos that role-play these styles.

Using a Style That Works

If you haven't guessed by now, the most effective form of communicating is being assertive. Yet according to experts, it's the one we use the least, which explains the great number of assertiveness training seminars that tens of thousands of people flock to every year. It also explains the great degree of conflict families face under the stress and challenges of caregiving.

On most personality and communication style surveys, I come out as assertive (and I confess, I've attended those seminars). I've been brought in by opposing groups to help facilitate compromises, and I enjoy the give-and-take of negotiating and discovering what motivates each side. I like helping them find mutual interests that lead them down a path toward a win-win solution.

But one day when it came to having a reasoned conversation with my 96-year-old grandmother-in-law, Lena, with vascular dementia, many of those skills went right out the window after she accused me of stealing her money. It was following a night of little sleep, due in part to my providing 'round-the-clock care for both her and my newborn. Lena had also become incontinent. Her dementia was mild, and even though, as an expert, I knew her paranoia was induced by a brain starved for oxygen and layered with proteins that sabotaged her thought processes, her accusation struck a nerve. I saw red. In a flash, I was behaving as an aggressive communicator. I slammed Lena's checkbook onto the dresser, saying, "Fine, then—I won't handle your money anymore." It wasn't one of my finer moments.

After I took a break, I returned to Lena's room, apologized, and asked her what worried her most about her money. Turns out, Lena had always feared that people were stealing from her. She was worried that the new clothes and supplies I had bought for her were using up all her money (they were actually gifts from us), and that would mean "there would be nothing left to bury me." Her greatest fear was not having a respectable funeral. Who knew? If we hadn't had that conversation, I never would have learned this about her and would have remained angry and unappreciated.

The dynamics between Lena and me could have become the perfect storm for a passive-aggressive way of communicating that neither one of us deserved. I share this story to illustrate that even though you may gravitate toward a productive style of communicating, factors of stress, fatigue, pressure, and raw emotions make us subject to using communication styles that can set us back and make us feel pretty lousy.

I know you don't have the time to run out to one of those stirring assertiveness training seminars, so let me share the best nuggets of advice from the experts on how to communicate in an assertive way to successfully guide your caregiving conversations.

Assess the communication style that the person you are speaking with is using. If the person is acting aggressive or passive-aggressive, don't respond in kind. Stay calm. Focus objectively on the issue in front of you. If the person is passive, gently encourage him to express his thoughts on what to do. Start with a small item to discuss, to build confidence; then move toward more difficult issues as the person feels more comfortable sharing his views.

Validate your understanding of what a person has said, especially, if it has been an emotionally charged exchange. Say something like, "Mom, let me make sure I hear what you're saying. You think that Dad has been under a lot of stress lately, which makes him flustered, and that's why he's been acting confused." Notice you're not saying that she's wrong or that she's ignoring the situation. You are objectively repeating the facts and your observation of what she has presented.

Use "I-statements." For example, say, "I'm worried about Dad's confusion, and I think there might be something more serious going on in addition to the stress. I think, for Dad's sake, it would be helpful for him to see his doctor, just to make sure."

Components of an "I-Statement"

An "I-statement" has four components:

- State exactly what was said or done that triggered your feelings.

- State the feelings you have.

- Explain why you feel the way you do.

- If appropriate, make a request stating what you need.

Source: Dr. Robert Nielson, North Dakota State University

In this example, you have met all four components of the "I-statement":

- You've explained what was done. (Dad has been acting confused.)

- You've explained how that made you feel. (You're worried.)

- You've explained why you feel this way. (It could be a sign that something more serious is going on.)

- You've explained that you're making a request to meet a need. (Dad needs to see his doctor.)

In addition, you have validated your mom's reasoning that stress has something to do with his confusion. But you are also clarifying why you are worried—you think there's more than just stress involved, yet you are not discounting it. This leaves the door open for a discussion that you both could be right about. You're headed for a win-win solution, especially for Dad, because his needs remain the focus of both of your concerns.

In contrast, avoiding "I-statements" would have resulted in a conversation like this: "Mom, *you* think that the only thing going on with Dad is just stress. *You* aren't seeing what I'm seeing. In fact, *you* are too close to him to see what's really going on." Now your mom needs to defend herself, and you've inferred that she's not as concerned as you are, which will make her feel personally attacked. She might lash back with, "*You* aren't here all the time—I know him better than *you,* and *you're* just blowing things out of proportion."

Most people become defensive when a sentence starts with *you*—it signals that they may need to defend themselves. A simple example is saying, "I think this is unfair" and then stating why you feel this way, as opposed to saying, "You're unfair."

Use body language that signals you care and are invested in what the other person is saying. Act confident, even when you're not, by keeping your posture upright, yet leaning forward just enough to show you are engaged without appearing aggressive. Nod your head as the other person speaks to show that you understand what's being said; use facial expressions that show you're interested; and avoid gesturing, making faces, or rolling your eyes when you disagree.

Use a calm, reassuring tone of voice when you speak. If things start to get emotional and are about to trigger a response that will get you off track, take a deep breath, relax for 10 seconds, and then respond. If you need more time, take a break.

Pushing Emotional Buttons

"The reason parents are so good at pushing your buttons is because they installed them!"

—Quote from a family caregiver who's been trying to "uninstall" a few

Rehearse what you want to say before going into a tough situation, to help you anticipate and keep your emotions in check. You'll be ready for any labeling and accusations if arguments start flying. Play out how you'll respond assertively, given the usual scenarios that come up in your family.

Never call people names ("You're lazy"), exaggerate ("I'm the only one who cares"), label people ("You're Daddy's Little Girl"), assign blame ("This is your fault"), threaten ("If you don't listen to me, I'm not coming back to visit or help you"), or make demands that induce fear or exploit dependency. Quite simply, play fair. Follow the basic principles of assertiveness:

- Be tactful and honest.

- Care about other people's feelings, but don't let them exploit or dominate you.

- Be willing to address potential misunderstandings before they fester.

- Respect and value each person.

- Regard other people's rights as you do your own.

- Set honest and reasonable limits on what you can do for someone instead of misleading them, no matter how well intentioned you are.

- Recognize that problem solving is an inclusive process by involving those who have a stake in its solution.

- Communicate openly.

- Accept that you are not responsible for other people's emotions.

- Finally, remember that it's okay to say no.

Being assertive takes practice and an inner awareness of yourself and others. Be patient with yourself, but do find ways to practice the principles of assertiveness every day so that it becomes second nature to you. Being assertive not only will improve your family life, but it also will empower you to become an effective advocate for your parent's health care, caregiving, and well-being.

Essential Takeaways

- We tend to prefer one communication style over another, but given certain circumstances, we use any of the basic four: passive, aggressive, passive-aggressive, or assertive.

- Our communication styles evolve from childhood through adulthood, honed from what's worked and what hasn't in our everyday exchanges with others. It's a work-in-progress at any age.

- Caregiving issues are often complex and require a great deal of open, honest, and collaborative communication—a tall order, given what's at stake and the stress those conversations often evoke.

- Practicing assertive communication means being authentic to yourself and others. It is the most healthy and productive form of communicating.

chapter 17

Four Classic Elder Care Conflicts

When it's time for Dad to retire from driving

When it's no longer safe for Mom to live alone

When your spouse doesn't want your parent to move in

What to do when you are feeling alone in caring for your parents when siblings don't share the caregiving load

Over the past 10 years, I've been writing a column, called "Our Parents, Ourselves," for a pretty wide readership. I've received loads of emails and letters from family members as they struggle with caring for each other. Busy lives, demands of family and careers, child rearing, unresolved conflicts, differences of opinion, and long distances all converge to make caregiving a rather tough undertaking.

Despite the wide range of questions I receive, four classic caregiving dilemmas repeatedly appear in my mailbox and may resonate with you as well. Hopefully, you'll gain some insights from my answers to them to make your experiences go a bit more smoothly.

Unsafe Drivers Who Won't Give Up the Keys

Thousands of families struggle with this issue every day. Driving is seen as every American's right, and an older driver's independence is largely based upon his or her ability to drive. Men, especially, become quite depressed when they are forced to give up the car keys; for them, a bit of their identity is caught up in their cars.

But driving isn't a right; it's a privilege. If your father is no longer a safe driver and is at significant risk of harming himself or others, your goal is to convince him to "retire" from driving, just like he retired from work. In fact, it's helpful to use the term *retire* instead of asking him to "give up his keys" or "quit" driving.

You might want to try one more conversation in trying to reason with your dad. Ask him to describe what he thinks life will be like when he does retire from driving in the *future*. Try to get him to describe the limitations he imagines will occur. Perhaps he can talk about how life changed for any of his friends who retired from driving.

This will give you insights into what motivates him to drive and what obstacles you'll need to address when he does retire from driving. If you can assure him that he can remain independent and stay active, he might be more inclined to let go. Many older people become depressed when they stop driving because it is a huge signal to their psyche that they are declining.

If your dad hasn't responded to age-related reasons to retire from driving (for example, vision impairment, loss of neck flexibility, and inability to multitask), approach him with financial and liability reasons. For example, you could suggest that he increase his liability limits on his auto insurance; if he injures someone, the medical bills could easily exceed his coverage and make him vulnerable to losing all his savings and property. Or show him the costs of driving every year (such as insurance, registration fees, maintenance, and gas). Even if he used a taxicab, he would still save money without limiting his ability to get around.

But if all else fails, here are two more strategies: Nearly all state Departments of Transportation provide steps for physicians and family members to report a driver who has exhibited diminished capacity that impairs driving ability due to some health condition. You could approach your father's primary care physician and report your concerns, along with any traffic citations, accident reports, fender benders, and unexplained dents that warrant intervention.

Encourage the doctor to talk with your dad. If he is still unwilling to retire from driving, ask the doctor to write a prescription for a voluntary driver's assessment.

Tip

You can find a local "Driver Rehabilitation Specialist" at www.aded.net, or call 1-877-529-1860. You will likely need to pay for the service.

If your father refuses this approach, then ask the physician to refer him to the Medical Review Board of your state's motor vehicle agency (Department of Transportation). If his doctor declines taking this action and you believe your father is a safety threat, you can make a referral. Most Departments of Transportation will want your name to verify that the report is not a prank, but they will keep your referral anonymous.

The majority of states throughout the nation (62 percent as of 2011) do not require older drivers to renew their licenses more often than other age groups. But as more older drivers remain on the road (more than half of people 85 years and older are licensed), many states are imposing accelerated license renewals. For example, Arizona, Colorado, Georgia, North Carolina, and South Carolina require those in their 60s to renew their license every five years. Illinois requires it every two years for drivers age 81 to 86 years.

The bottom line is that every state has its own (if any) older driver restrictions. To learn about your state's policies and laws, go to the Insurance Institute for Highway Safety, at www.iihs.org, and, in the search bar, enter "older driver laws"—or go to your state's Department of Transportation for details.

You have every right to encourage your parent to retire from driving. Teens and drivers 74 years and older have the highest auto accident fatality rates in the country. Most of those accidents happen just a few miles from home. My rule of thumb is always that if you wouldn't allow your children in the car with your parent behind the wheel, why is Mom or Dad driving?

Tip

Your father can assess his driving skills on a home computer by way of a software program available as a CD-ROM from your local American Automobile Association (AAA) titled "Roadwise Review." You can also download it free from the AAA Foundation for Traffic Safety at www. seniordrivers.org. It measures eight functional abilities that predict crash risks among older drivers. "Roadwise Review" can help you assess: Leg Strength and General Mobility, Head/Neck Flexibility, High-Contrast Visual Acuity, Low-Contrast Visual Acuity, Working Memory, Visualization of Missing Information, Visual Search, and Useful Field of View.

When Dementia Makes Living Alone Unsafe

If none of the strategies we discussed on living alone in Chapter 7 is appropriate for your mother and she has undergone testing that's rendered a diagnosis of dementia, you really have no choice but to find an alternative solution to her living alone. It's a tough spot to be in—you don't want to traumatically remove her from her home, yet you feel irresponsible if you don't do something.

Because your mom has dementia, "reasoning" with her will be difficult because you don't share the same reality. Your most effective ally will be her primary care physician or the geriatrician who diagnosed her with Alzheimer's disease or other form of dementia.

Arrange an appointment with her doctor and ask to speak to him or her ahead of time. Explain that it's no longer safe for your mother to live alone and that you need assistance in convincing her that living alone is no longer in her best interest. Provide the doctor with a list of examples that shows she can no longer perform the tasks of daily living (use the list described in Chapter 3).

If she's had safety incidents, such as leaving the stove on, forgetting to lock doors, or wandering in the neighborhood, share that information as well. Also describe your family situation and let the doctor know that, as a family, you cannot provide the 24/7 supervision needed for her to remain at home.

Ask the doctor whether he could "prescribe" a week at a "center" for necessary treatment for her condition. If this is coming from her physician instead of her "interfering or overreactive" children, she might listen. If it's written as a prescription, your mother might be less resistant and might view taking this action as medical treatment, which might be more acceptable to her than seeming defeated by Alzheimer's.

If the doctor presents going to a center as a temporary measure, she might not feel like she's being backed into a corner. Also, if her sense of time has been affected, the "week" might easily transition into a permanent solution. Another way of easing her into the idea might be to ask those in charge of the facility if you could bring your mom for lunch and eat there as you would in any other restaurant.

Dr. Roger Cadieux, clinical professor of psychiatry at Penn State University, Hershey Medical Center, who practices adult and geriatric psychiatry, had this to say when I asked him how he would handle this situation: "The approach that I use is to sympathetically but firmly present the findings and then state definitely that there is now a need for a higher level of care. There is usually a great deal of distress, but the anger, if any, is directed toward the physician and not the family. I make sure that the patient understands that I am their advocate even though I am imparting difficult information. The challenge is for the family to find a physician who can and will take this approach."

Dr. Cadieux recommends giving your mother the opportunity to participate, if possible, in the process of finding a facility conducive to her needs. When warranted, he suggests that medication, especially low doses of antidepressants and/or antipsychotics, can make the difference between easy acceptance and abject refusal of this necessary and wise move.

Considering Your Spouse's Feelings When Your Parent Moving In Is Up for Discussion

Caregiving isn't a solo act, even if you aren't married or have no siblings. You'll always need to reach out for help. But when caregiving involves a spouse, it must be a partnership for your marriage to survive. So if your husband or wife is having second thoughts *before* your mom moves in, both of you need to thoughtfully and objectively consider all your options, review your mom's needs, and create a plan that includes finding ways to nurture your marriage along the way. Most moms don't want their son or daughter's marriage to come unglued over caring for them. So let's begin with the premise that taking care of your marriage is an integral part of taking care of your mom.

Remember in Chapter 3 when we went over conducting a caregiving inventory and then developed goals so that you could create workable solutions? Be sure to follow those same steps now.

One underlying question that should guide you as you consider different options and identify your mom's caregiving needs is whether having her live with you is in *her* best interest. Before you answer that question, refer back to Chapter 7's descriptions of a wide array of living options. When you've taken all those steps, you'll be in a much better position to know what direction to pursue.

If your husband or wife has shared doubts with you, let him or her express them without you becoming defensive. Don't let this spiral down to "It's your mom or me" or "Not allowing me to take care of my mother means you really don't love me." Hopefully by now, you and your spouse have learned how to reach a compromise.

Find a neutral or favorite place and hear your spouse out. Ask what worries him most. Encourage him to describe how he sees life living with your mother. Then you share your worries and how you see the future. Openly discuss how it might affect your marriage, even if your mom doesn't come to live with you. Would that make you grow resentful, leading him to feel guilty while both of your emotions turn into anger toward each other?

Again, go through the problem-solving steps so you'll know what solutions make the most sense for all of you. I can't stress this enough. Your mom, of course, should be part of the process.

<table>
<tr><td>MISC.</td></tr>
</table>

Consider Your Parent's Feelings

A move for your parent will go more smoothly and be more compassionate if you consider what Mom or Dad might be feeling:

- Sad about giving up home, friends, and community
- Defeated by failing health
- Anxious over being seen as a burden
- Fearful of becoming dependent on others
- Lonely and isolated from peers

Find ways to help your parent express these feelings and restore a sense of purpose, independence, and dignity within your home.

If you and your spouse ask your mother to live with you, here are some added suggestions for making it work:

1. Ask your mother to describe her daily routine and what matters most to her in retaining it. Share your routine and your spouse's, and identify ways you might need to accommodate each other. Come up with solutions now, before they become a problem.

2. Specify one evening a week when you and your spouse go out (as in, on a date). If your mother knows this ahead of time, she won't feel "left out" or rejected. You could also give her a gentle reminder by saying something like, "Mom, we're going to an event on Friday. Is there anything you need while we're gone?"

3. Talk openly with your mom about how she'll always be your mother, but you're not a kid anymore and you're also a spouse. Identify ways you can spend time together, yet set boundaries while you fulfill your other roles.

4. If your mom isn't a "joiner," you might need to bring people to meet her or take her to activities so she can make friends. Just like every other member of the family, she needs outside interests so that the household doesn't become her entire world.

5. How you design space in the house for your mother is extremely important. She needs to have her own domain so that she can respect the private spaces of other family members, too. For

example, she might enjoy having a small refrigerator and micro-wave for her snacks in her room, along with her own television. It should be a pleasant space and a personal refuge—something that every family member needs.

6. Finally, you, your spouse, and your mother need to discuss who is going to pay for what. All too often, finances become the light-ning rod for unresolved emotional conflicts. Even if the topic feels uncomfortable, do it now, before you're in the midst of a family feud. If siblings can contribute to certain expenses, get that out on the table now.

If your mother has high caregiving needs and/or suffers from dementia, the following are some added steps to take.

1. Make a plan for respite care. This isn't an option. If your mom can't be left safely alone during the day, find out whether your local Area Agency on Aging can help subsidize the costs of your mom attend-ing an adult day center three times a week. It will greatly aid her and give you time to work or simply take a break. If you have sib-lings, ask them to set aside weekends or even a week to come stay with your mother while you and your spouse get away. At the very least, arrange for help (such as a volunteer, family member, or paid caregiver) to relieve you during the week.

2. If you have siblings, share the list of caregiving needs you've cre-ated and ask them to sign up for what they can do. I recommend creating a Letter of Understanding so that everyone knows what's expected.

3. Definitely think through a Plan B to go into effect if your mother's health deteriorates. A time might come when her care is really beyond you and your spouse's ability. A geriatric care manager (see Chapter 6) can be a terrific resource to help you sort through your mom's needs, your resources, and the options available to you and your husband in providing her care.

Most people don't realize the extent to which caregiving affects their lives. Being realistic, learning to openly communicate, and thinking through your options will make it more likely that your multigenerational household will be something you treasure rather than regret.

Call your local Area Agency on Aging (Eldercare Locator: 1-800-677-1116) to see whether you qualify for the Family Caregiver Support Program.

Soliciting Help from Siblings When You're the Caregiver

Probably the most universal complaint among caregivers is the lack of dependable (if any) help from other family members. In the National Family Caregiver's Association annual survey, three out of four family members felt this way.

It's relatively common for one family member to gravitate to the central role of caregiver. Most often, it's the child who lives the closest to the parent. If everyone lives out of town, it might fall on the oldest child, the sibling with the most flexible work schedule, the one with grown children, or the sibling with a health background. So if you're a nurse without kids at home living closest to your parents, it's no contest who's going to be the caregiver.

Many caregivers fall into the same trap that I succumbed to when I cared for my grandmother-in-law who came to live with us. It didn't take long for Lena and me to get into a routine, and I began to feel like no one else could take care of her like I could. It was too much of a hassle to show another family member what to do or find reputable help. Lena also fed into this; she just wanted me to take care of her and affectionately called me her "manager." And so the cycle began. Just like so many other caregivers, I became worn down and resentful that others wouldn't help.

Many caregivers feel that other family members should just *know* what to do and pitch in voluntarily. They resent having to ask for help. But sending hints to your siblings or hoping they'll just "get it" isn't enough. Some of your siblings might think that you have everything under control. Or they might simply turn a blind eye and ignore the whole situation.

So let's give them some vision and a reality check. Most people don't realize how stressful caregiving is until they've gone through it, which means you need to create a picture of what it takes to care for your mom. Your siblings can't do their fair share if they don't get the whole picture. The best way to convey to them what's needed is to go over all the caregiving tasks your mother requires and the amount of time each takes by following the ADL and IADL lists presented in Chapter 3.

You'll then be in a position to sit down with your sibling(s) and share the lists. If your siblings don't get along, I recommend doing this with each one individually.

Instead of counting on a "look at what a martyr I am" approach to catapult them into guilt-ridden action, start by asking them to help you go through the list and provide input on how each of you can come up with a care plan for your mother. If a sibling lives some distance away, can he or she do things that don't involve being there? Perhaps your brother can handle all the insurance work and schedule doctor appointments, while your sister pays bills and helps research any of your mom's medical conditions. Could either of them set aside some time one day a week to relieve you of your caregiving tasks? If they can't, could they cover the costs of providing some assistance for that day? When it comes to gifts for Mom, suggest that they give gift certificates for home-delivered meals, cab rides, home-care aides, or a cleaning service—all of which would assist you as well.

When you've developed a care plan with their input, make copies of it and treat it as a working document to reference and update as your mother's circumstances change. I also recommend setting up a weekly phone call to go over your mother's care—that way, your siblings will feel more invested and remain aware of your mother's ever-evolving needs. Start relating to your siblings as partners; hopefully, they'll return the favor.

If Your Sibling Doesn't Get Along with Your Parent

If you're caught up in a situation in which, for example, your brother doesn't get along with your dad, whom you're taking care of, and he uses that as the reason not to help, you need to reframe the question of "Who needs the care?" At first blush, it seems like the answer is your father, and that allows your brother to rationalize why it's not his responsibility to help pitch in.

All siblings have a different relationship with each of their parents. Regrettably, sometimes those relationships are like broken glass, with shards of anger and wounded feelings from years past. In those instances, even if a sibling has tried offering the care, the parent might refuse it or make insulting remarks during the process. On the other hand, the adult child could be the one hurling insults, and the dependent parent feels victimized by the experience. Either way, it's not a healthy scenario—and you aren't the one responsible for fixing it.

So let's return to that question, "Who needs the care?" The answer is you. The goal is to get your brother to refocus and realize that the one in need is his sister, with whom he does have a relationship worth preserving. Instead of getting into a debate over whether he should forgive your father, make amends, or decide who is right or wrong, let's take a look at what steps you can take.

First, share that caregiving task list you created as a result of "working toward solutions," in Chapter 3. But this time, redefine it and pull from the list the items that *you* need help with and that don't involve direct contact with your father.

Second, approach your brother in a positive way—no guilt-tripping him or making him feel that you're the superior child because you're the caregiver. You might say something like, "I'm starting to find that caring for Dad is affecting (whatever it is) and that I'm just not able to keep up with by myself. I understand that you feel that Dad wouldn't want your help, and I appreciate why you feel that way. Yet there are ways that you can help me, and it won't even involve Dad directly. I could sure use a brother." Then give him an opening to respond. Hopefully, he'll ask how he can help.

Ways Your Sibling Can Help Without Interacting with Your Parent

Share the caregiving tasks you've been performing that do not involve direct interaction with your parent, like scheduling doctor's appointments, handling the paperwork, or making meals that could be dropped off at your place or a neighbor's. Your sibling could make calls to the local Area Agency on Aging (1-800-677-1116 or www.eldercare.gov) and other agencies, to see whether your parent qualifies for benefits and services. Or he or she could go online at www.benefitscheckup.org.

You both could decide that it might make sense to share the costs of having someone come over and perform some of the tasks that you are currently doing. Nonmedical senior care companies can do many caregiver tasks and even provide companionship to your parent. You'll find them in the Yellow Pages, usually under "Home Care Agencies" or "Home Health" (such as Comfort Keepers, Visiting Angels, and Home Instead Senior Care).

Hopefully, this approach allows your sibling to become a partner in your caregiving. Just remember to keep the focus on you. Even if your brother or sister says something like, "But Dad hates me and I really don't like him—why should I help?" remain calm. Reassure your sibling that you understand how difficult this can be.

If you continue to be the sole caregiver, it is far more likely that your relationship with your sibling will become strained and perhaps just as broken as it is with your parent. Caregiving is stressful, and it won't take long before you feel resentful that it's all on your shoulders. You deserve your sibling's support, and he or she deserves being asked to give it.

Essential Takeaways

- Driving is a privilege, not a right. If your parent is clearly an unsafe driver and you've tried unsuccessfully to convince him or her that it's time to retire, either reach out to a physician to prescribe a driving assessment or pursue your state's steps to report an unsafe driver.

- Your family physician can be an ally in convincing patients with dementia that the time has come to receive more comprehensive care at a facility rather than live alone.

- Bringing in a parent to live with you can be rewarding, but if you are married, remember that caregiving is a partnership. Your spouse must be part of the decision making from the beginning. If there are children in the household, their feelings must be considered, too.

- Caregiving is a family affair when siblings are involved. Even if they live out of town, they can perform certain tasks and need to be asked to assist. Beware of the "I'd rather do it myself" trap.

chapter 18

Talking Through Money Issues

The real costs of elder care

Appreciating your parent's desire for legacy

How money styles can confound caregiving issues

Setting up a caregiving budget to save time, money, and headaches

Money matters are rarely simple when it comes to caregiving. Parents and their children might avoid talking about them because the issues they bring up cause feelings of discomfort. But given the costs of elder care and the likelihood that your parent will need various levels of it, the topic deserves your attention, patience, and due diligence.

Understanding you, your sibling's, and parent's money style is the first step in initiating a conversation on the financial aspects of your parent's care. Given the complex emotions that many of us feel about money, you're better off having that "money talk" long before your back is up against a wall. Let's look at ways to plan, talk, and act when addressing the costs associated with caring for your parents.

Why You Should Talk About Money: The Costs of Elder Care

What comes to most people's minds when they hear "long-term care" or "elder care" is the cost of a nursing home. They know it's expensive, and that is surely true, but many people also assume that either Medicare or the state will cover it.

And that's one mighty wrong calculation. Medicare, the federal health insurance program, may cover up to 100 skilled nursing days under certain limitations. But that's it. On the state side of the equation, people who are impoverished might qualify for Medicaid, but they will have "spent down" their assets before they qualify. So if they had a life savings, they've depleted it. If you think you can quickly transfer your mom or dad's savings and assets to meet the low-income eligibility threshold of the state, you can't. "Look-back" laws require that a person's assets for up to five years prior to applying for state welfare (Medicaid) count toward his or her income.

Nursing home care is the most costly of all long-term care services, due to the nature of 'round-the-clock skilled nursing care provided to residents. If your parent is 85 years and older, the likelihood of him or her needing nursing home care greatly increases. In fact, 14.3 percent of older Americans in this age group live in a nursing home. Half of them can expect to live there for a year, and one in five will reside at the facility for almost five years.

And what's the price tag for a nursing home stay? The national median for a one-year stay is $77,745 or $193 per day for a semiprivate room, according to Genworth's 2011 Cost of Care Survey. Those are daunting numbers for any American family.

Tip

According to the AARP Public Policy Institute, nearly two thirds of Americans over age 65 will need long-term care at home, through adult day health care, or in an assisted living facility or nursing home.

Most people try to avoid being placed in a nursing home. Over the past decade, a wide range of options and services have developed in response to the growth of the older population, states shifting their budgets away from nursing homes and toward community-based care, and people simply wanting to "age in place." In other words, they want to stay home.

Most of the services that make it possible for you to care for your loved one at home or in the community will be coming out of your parent's pockets—and possibly yours. The Genworth Cost Study also found that when an older person suffers a long-term care event (such as a specific illness, age-related frailty, or dementia), that person will spend about $14,000 for care, and family members will contribute an average of $8,000 in out-of-pocket expenses. Savings and retirement contributions are the first to succumb, placing your parents in a precarious position to meet the care demands of likely episodes down the road.

For an idea of how those expenses add up, take a look at the National Median Rates for the following services:

Elder Care Service	National Median Rate
Homemaker (cooking, errands)	$18 per hour
Home health aide (bathing, dressing)	$19 per hour
Adult day center (therapeutic activities)	$60 per day
Assisted living (S/O, one B/R)	$3,261 per month

Source: Genworth Cost Study 2011

Based on these figures, assisted living would cost your parent $39,100 per year—and that doesn't include home health aide services or any form of nursing care. Let's say your dad has a financial portfolio of $500,000 and chooses to live in assisted living. That amount would last less than 13 years, and that's just covering the rent. If he entered assisted living in his early 70s, by the time he reached his mid-80s, his financial resources would be depleted. Before you panic, review the resources available for your parents in Chapter 6, especially the public caregiving programs.

It's Not Just About the Money

Nearly every therapist who works with couples or families arguing over money will tell you that it really isn't about the money. It's about so much more. How we view money, handle it, spend it, save it, or squander it is all wrapped up in how we view ourselves and what money symbolizes to us. Understanding your personal relationship with money and how it influences the decisions you make regarding your parent's care is a critical step toward preventing caregiving money conflicts with your parent and other family members.

The most frequent financial complaint I receive from family caregivers is not over how much money parents spend on elder care or services—it's how *little*. Adult children find it exasperating when they believe their parents are placing their health and safety at risk because they won't spend money that they do have.

To make the point, here's Maggie's story: Maggie was especially upset with her recently widowed mom, who wouldn't pay $48 a month for a personal alert system. Her mother now lives alone and has no one close by who would hear her call for help. Her mother, who could easily afford the device, saw it as a waste of money, but her daughter viewed it as wise: "Doesn't she realize how much more it will cost if she hurts herself and can't get immediate help? She could be having a stroke, and because no one helped her in time, she could be spending the rest of her life in a nursing home. Then *all* of her money would be gone!"

Maggie's mother may have turned down the use of a personal alert system for a host of reasons. Yes, it could be as simple as believing she couldn't afford it, but she also might have viewed wearing one of the devices as a badge of vulnerability and old age.

A powerful motivator is at play among older parents that adult children may not fully appreciate. It's about legacy. Their parents are at a stage in their lives in which creating and leaving a legacy is very important to them.

Many in our parents' generation evaluate a "life well lived" based on how much wealth they are able to leave to their children. It symbolizes that they saved, worked hard, and were able to provide for their family. The desire to leave an inheritance that reinforces feelings of self-worth may overpower decisions to spend money on themselves—even when it's in their best interest. That's not what's driving your parent's money-related decisions right now.

The Value of Money

"When you turn toward your money and begin to value it, nurture it, and truly respect it for what it can (and cannot) do, you will understand that the true value of money is the value you give it."

—Suze Orman, *Money Cards, Words That Lead to Wealth*

So even when you and your siblings tell your mom or dad, "We really don't care about an inheritance—we'd rather you take care of yourself," the message won't resonate. In fact, you may be insulting them, all while you see yourself as being generous and looking out for them.

Another frequent motivator that prevents older parents from spending money on elder care is that they can't see paying someone to do the chores and daily living tasks they've always done, even when it ensures their safety, health, and quality of life. For starters, they often don't recognize that they need such services. In addition, unlike their baby boomer children, they haven't been hiring caterers, gardeners, child care, home cleaning services, or Mr. Fix-It for simple home repairs, or calling for take-out to feed the kids at the end of a long day.

The older generation, which might not appreciate the juggling act between career and family that their adult children perform, views these chores as something that parents, friends, and relatives do. They can't imagine the need for a stranger to come into their homes and help them cook, shop, pay bills, remind them to take pills, or assist them with getting in and out of chairs or taking a shower. Again, in their mind, it's a waste of money chipping away at their legacy.

Even if you try to pay for these services, you may run into resistance. In their mind, it's still a waste of money. The only way I convinced my father to accept using a personal emergency response system (PERS) was to say that his health plan covered it. But truth be told, the "health plan" is an automatic deduction from my checking account. The sales associate who arranges for a national company selling PERS told me, "I can't tell you how many adult children are paying for their parent's system and telling them it's covered by Medicare. It's the only way they'll accept using it."

What's Your Money Style?

Because at some time you're going to have discussions involving money with your parents and other family members, let's take some time to review your own personal money style. If you've ever read books by or listened to award-winning personal finance advisor Suze Orman, you've learned that views about money are formed from personal experiences and memories from childhood.

Money Memories

"Messages about money are passed down from generation to generation, worn and chipped like family dishes. Your own memories about money will tell you a lot, if you take a step back and see how those memories influenced who you were—and whether those memories still influence who you are today."

—Suze Orman, *Financial Guidebook, Put the 9 Steps to Work, 2nd Edition*

Maybe your parents taught you that money is the root of all evil, or that it's impolite to talk about money, or ingrained in you the saying, "Never a borrower or lender be." You may have heard your parents argue over money, or you grew up feeling embarrassed that you had less than your friends. It might be helpful to step back in time and recall your childhood memories of money, especially as they relate to what your parents taught you. Doing so will provide insights on your conversations with them about money matters and roadblocks you may experience regarding elder care expenses.

Now let's fast-forward to your current age and look at four basic money styles that experts commonly describe. Most people have a tendency toward one particular style yet exhibit traits of all four in certain situations. Which ones resonate the most with you?

The Saver

Here's someone who values money, wants to keep it safe, and loves finding ways to get more of it, especially hunting down a great bargain. They can't resist coupons, and they love setting up a budget and sticking to it. Savers usually have a hard time spending money on themselves or loved ones because they are more concerned with having money in the future than having it in the present.

Deep down, they worry that they may outlive their assets. Because they've taken control over their money, chances are good that they'll want to control all of the family's finances. The Savers' attraction to detail can blind them from the big picture and may make loved ones feel slighted or annoyed. Their self-esteem is caught up in how much money they've saved. Sometimes you'll see the term *hoarder* associated with this style.

The Spender

Friends out for a good time and credit card companies sure love spenders. They listen to an inner voice that tells them they deserve that designer dress, the luxury car, and a home they likely can't afford. They often shower family and friends with gifts, making the spenders feel loved and respected—in fact, it's how many Spenders gain a sense of self-worth. They enjoy living in the moment and follow the mantra, "You only go around once." Some spenders have the money to spend, but many are counting on a rescue fantasy to get them out of debt. Some spenders go on binges or splurges, spending excessive amounts of money that they later regret.

The Avoider

Balancing a checkbook, maintaining a savings account, paying bills, investing, and working within a budget just aren't worth the time or effort for Avoiders. But underneath that *laissez-faire* attitude, Avoiders may also feel anxious about money and would rather ignore what they really feel.

Some believe that money is the "root of all evil," so focusing on it means they are greedy and betraying their spiritual values. Others lack confidence in money matters, so they avoid financial planning at all costs. And costly it is: few avoiders have a retirement income to carry them through old age.

MISC.

A Nation of Avoiders?

More than 90 percent of participants in a national Age Wave/Harris Interactive survey reported that, even though they worry about becoming a burden to their family, they haven't had a conversation with loved ones about potential long-term care expenses, the costs of care, or what they would prefer if they need it.

The Worrier

Most of us have money worries at some time, but Worriers fret constantly even when they have enough money in the bank and have just paid their bills. They worry about running out of money and often second-guess every purchase or financial decision they make. Worriers find themselves paralyzed in making financial choices because they worry they'll make the wrong one. Their anxieties may stem from feeling a lack of confidence, from being compulsive or being a perfectionist, or from growing up in a household where their parents openly expressed their money worries—real or imagined.

If you see any resemblance to yourself, your siblings, or your parents in these profiles, you might get a few hints to how your money style influences the choices you make and recommend regarding your parent's elder care. Now let's look at how these styles play out in the world of caregiving.

Talking Through Money and Elder Care Issues

It helps to know that each money style has advantages and disadvantages. So rather than view your parents, spouse, or siblings at opposite ends when your styles aren't the same, identify ways in which they can complement each other.

For example, imagine that your recently widowed mother, who lives alone, can't drive, and uses a walker, is pondering whether to move to a senior living community. The community offers independent apartments, transportation, assisted living, and home health aide services. Your sister, who is a spender, thinks it's a great idea because she wants Mom to be more active and make friends. She figures she'll have enough money to live there once she sells the house, so why not just go with it?

But you're a saver, and a bit of a worrier, too, so you think it's really important to weigh the pros and cons and do a cost-benefit analysis. You want to know how long Mom's money will last and exactly what the monthly fees will cover. Your mom is an avoider, and she has always let your father handle the finances. Now she's looking to you, her son, to do the same.

Instead of arguing with your sister over "what's best for Mom," you could use your differing perspectives to cover all the bases in exploring your mom's options. Before you take this action, review the problem-solving strategies outlined in Chapters 2 and 3; your first step is deciding what "problem" the move solves.

When you've determined that moving to a senior living community solves problems that your mom needs and wants to fix, parcel out who analyzes what, given your money style.

In this instance, your sister could take your mom to view different places, but the agreement is that she will bring back all of the "fine print" language and literature that details the contracts and fees. Your sister and mom's job is to make a list of the pros and cons of each place in terms of lifestyle factors such as social interaction, mobility, physical exercise, and nutritious meals at the dining room. Your job is to identify the actual costs of living there and any pitfalls in contract language and fees that would jeopardize your mom's financial reserve. You and your sister could divvy up the research on quality markers of each senior living community (see Chapter 7).

All three of you could develop "what if" scenarios (see Chapter 4) so you can cost out what would happen if your mom needed more hands-on care and moved into an assisted living facility, or if she remained in an independent apartment but hired home care aides to help.

This type of exercise uses everyone's strengths—it allows the saver/worrier to see intangible lifestyle benefits and the big picture, the spender can see the real and actual costs of choosing various living arrangements, and the avoider can learn to engage in a financial conversation to express her living preferences, some of which she may never have had vocalized or realized. If your mom avoids talking about money because it worries her, then working out a plan with her son and daughter that specifies where the money to care for her will come from will save her sleepless nights in her new digs.

A Few More Financial Considerations

Plenty of books have been written on financial planning and how people relate to money. Finance books targeting baby boomers mostly focus on how to plan for their retirement. Hopefully, after realizing what the costs of long-term care can do to your nest egg, you'll be more inclined to assess your own finances and take steps to protect them in case you need elder care sooner than planned. Yet adult children need to know more about elder care finances than planning solely for their own retirement.

Tip

Given today's blended and extended families, you may find yourself caring not only for your parents, but also for your in-laws and step-parents. Some of you will also care for your parent's new partner following a divorce or death, and that will include learning to work with a whole new set of extended family members you hardly even know.

Beyond what we've already discussed, here are some more tips when dealing with elder care and finances:

- **Think about the financial impact before quitting a job.** If you're thinking about leaving your job to care for a loved one, it's vital that you consider the financial impact this will have, not only on losing a paycheck in the short run, but also on your future earning potential if you ever want to re-enter the job market. Will it affect vesting requirements that would earn you benefits such as pensions, bonuses, or pay for accumulated vacation days? What amount of loss will you bear if you no longer receive 401(k) employer contributions or paid health insurance? You may decide that other options, such as a reverse mortgage of your parent's home, make more sense. Some families pull together and draft a caregiving contract to basically employ a family member who is willing to quit a job and provide care. I recommend asking an elder care lawyer to draft such an agreement to ensure peace in the family.

- **Talk to your employer.** You may be surprised at what companies offer their employees today, in recognition of the growing demands elder care places on the workforce. Ask about flex time; see if they'll help pay for the services of a geriatric care manager (GCM) to help you sort through your loved one's care; and ask how you can piece together vacation days, sick leave, and family medical leave when you unexpectedly need to care for your parent. If your job offers long-term care insurance as a benefit for you, seriously consider it.

- **Track your caregiving expenses.** Making informed decisions on what elder care services or living arrangements make the most sense requires a realistic assessment of both the human and financial cost of care. Most people underestimate both; to gain a true picture of the costs, create a caregiving budget that identifies all the expenses— those that you and other family members contribute to and those your parent does. This should also include factors such as travel cost, lost wages, and any out-of-pocket expenses you incur.

- **Unlock the legacy hold.** If inheritance is the driving force behind your mother's reluctance to spend money on her care or services, look for a few compromises on how she can afford the care while still being able to provide for a reasonable inheritance. Consider you and your siblings sharing some of the costs now, knowing that the inheritance will likely replenish some of those expenditures later. It might also be beneficial for your mother to better understood how the costs associated with *not* receiving needed services and care jeopardize the savings that she so proudly cherishes.

- **Check into tax deductions for dependent care.** If you cover more than half of your parent's costs for housing, food, transportation, medical care, and other necessary living expenses, you may be able to claim your parent as a dependent. Your parent does not need to live with you to be declared your dependent. Your parent's income must be under a certain limit set each year by the IRS, which does not include Social Security income. Your parent must, however, include income from pension benefits, interest and dividends from investments, or withdrawals from any retirement savings plans, like IRAs. Even if your parent doesn't qualify as a dependent, other deductions for medical expenses might apply. For more information, see IRS Publication 502, on medical and dental expenses; talk to a tax accountant; or call Eldercare Locator, at 1-800-677-1116, to find a State Health Insurance Program (SHIP) volunteer advisor near you.

- **Watch out for scams.** Regretfully, scam artists prey on older people who have good credit and are trusting. An estimated 14,000 illegal telemarketing operations fleece at least $40 billion out of unsuspecting Americans every year. More than half of the victims are among the elderly. The National Fraud Information Center, run by the National Consumer League, warns that your parents might be a target if they are:

    - Receiving loads of junk mail for contests, "free trips," prizes, and sweepstakes.

    - Receiving frequent calls from strangers who promise valuable awards, great moneymaking deals, or requests for charitable contributions.

    - Having payments picked up by a private "courier" service.

    - Receiving lots of cheap items (prizes), such as costume jewelry, beauty products, or small appliances. In some cases, your parent might have bought these to supposedly win a bigger prize.

    - Receiving calls from organizations that say they will recover money (for a fee) that your parent paid to a telemarketer.

If you see these warning signs, don't blame your parents or make them feel foolish. If you do, they may fear that if they tell you everything, you might take away their financial control. Instead, let them know that you suspect something and that these people might be taking advantage of their honest, polite, and trusting nature.

Tip

If you're not sure whether it's a scam, counselors will help you sort this out at the National Fraud Information Center. Call 1-800-876-7060 or file an online incident report at www.fraud.org. You also can call your state's Office of the Attorney General, as most have a consumer hotline.

Not every parent is comfortable talking about money matters, yet it's such an important discussion to engage. Here are a couple more strategies to get it started:

- One way of broaching the topic of money with parents who tend to ignore it is to mention it casually by relating stories of friends who faced circumstances similar to theirs and took certain steps to protect their finances. Or reference an article you've read or financial-planning steps you've taken that will better secure your future. If they have mentioned wanting to do something for their grandchildren, use that as an opportunity to explore their portfolio options that include covering elder care expenses.

- Seek professional advice from elder law lawyers and financial planners so that your parents make sound and accurate decisions. If your family is at an impasse or can't negotiate financial issues, find a mediator, such as a GCM or social worker.

After my mother-in-law died from breast cancer, she left a handwritten note to my husband and his sister and attached it to her will, "If you treat your money as a friend, it will be a friend in return."

What a lovely note and a legacy.

Essential Takeaways

- Given the high likelihood that caregiving events will cost sizable amounts of money, having a calm conversation on how to finance it lays the groundwork for sound decisions when a crisis hits.

- We all have different money styles that have emotional underpinnings. The trick is to understand those emotions and appreciate how different styles can complement each other.

- Leaving a legacy through an inheritance is a powerful factor that influences the choices your parents make regarding how and what they will spend their money on during this life stage.

- Before you begin arguing over money, take the time to listen for the underlying message and what's really going on.

chapter 19

Talking Through Dementia

The effect of dementia on family members

Avoiding the pain of "reading into" hurtful outbursts

Your loved one's capacity to still care deeply about certain values

Effectively talking to someone with dementia

"Having a life," even when life is different

Caring for someone with dementia is probably one of the most trying experiences family members will ever endure. Many have likened it to being in a state of perpetual mourning. Family members watch their loved one suffer a cascade of losses, and they mourn each one of them. They grieve over a future neither of them will come to know. Perhaps the greatest loss is the day a spouse of 50 years becomes a stranger, as does a beloved daughter or son.

Amid this sea of loss is an island of refuge that many caregivers reach. They find meaning and purpose in their caregiving, especially for older spouses. Many of them have retired and find a renewed sense of purpose in their lives by caring for their spouse. Adult children view it as an opportunity to give back to parents who, in most cases, devotedly raised them.

Despite all the good intentions, caring for someone with dementia is fraught with stress that can be both physically and mentally draining.

And it won't be a short stint. According to the National Alzheimer's Association, dementia caregivers are likely to provide care for five years and more. Most people survive an average of 4 to 8 years after an Alzheimer's diagnosis, whereas some live up to 20 years with the disease.

Before you read this chapter, I suggest that you go back to Chapter 1 for a brief recap on the physiological effects of dementia. Even if your parent doesn't have dementia, much of the advice on how to relate and the core values of care receivers are worth a quick read.

Family Emotions

Although family members might not reach the conclusion at the same time, most will suspect that a loved one has Alzheimer's or another form of dementia before a physician ever renders a diagnosis.

In fact, 9 out of 10 do, according to a survey of 1,000 family caregivers by the National Alliance for Caregivers. But once that official diagnosis is given, families can expect to be hit with a wave of emotions. During the early stages, you, your parent, and your siblings might feel some or all of the emotional reactions I'm about to describe.

Sadness and Depression

When the reality of the diagnosis sets in, family members begin to understand the profound impact the disease will have on their relationship with their loved one. It will undoubtedly change, and there will be losses associated with it. For a spouse, it is particularly difficult because roles, routines, and endearing ways of communicating with each other will be altered.

You might feel sad for yourself because of the changes and losses, sad for the person with dementia, and sad for your healthy parent. This sadness can turn into depression. One of the most consistent findings from every survey taken of caregivers reveals high levels of depression. Forty to 70 percent of caregivers exhibit clinical symptoms of depression, and 25 percent meet the diagnostic criteria for major depression.

Anxiety, Anger, and Guilt

Losing a loved one to Alzheimer's or any other form of dementia can quickly lead to anxiety because the future is such an unknown commodity. You're not quite sure how your loved one will progress with the disease. Even though there are stages and professionals can advise you on what to expect, each person's dementia is unique to his or her brain and personality. Your family might also worry about the financial consequences of caring for your loved one and the new roles and responsibilities that different members will need to assume.

All these concerns can prompt a strong dose of anxiety. They can also provoke anger. It might start with "why" questions. Why your loved one? Why your family? Why you? You might worry that the disease is genetic and that it might be in your future as well. For example, as you begin caring for your mom, you might become angry at her behavior when she says or does something that's irritating or when she acts ungrateful for your care. And you might feel angry with other family members for not doing their "fair" share.

Sometimes you'll express your anger in ways that you regret, which will spark emotions of guilt. The anger and anxiety are normal, as are feelings of guilt. You will need to work through these potentially toxic emotions so that you don't let them dominate your caregiving and dictate how you relate to your family.

Embarrassment and Isolation

Some family members feel ashamed about the diagnosis and try to protect the loved one from embarrassing social situations. It's not unusual during the early stages for family members to "cover up" for the loved one—they'll volunteer a missing word when Mom can't find the right one to express what she wants to say, for example, or they'll divert attention away from Dad's diminished social skills.

Because caregivers find it stressful to take their loved one to social settings, they start declining invitations to go out. For the healthy spouse, this can become isolating and lead to feelings of loneliness. It can also make the disease progress more quickly. Social stimulation from interacting with people and engaging in activities that exercise thinking skills is extremely valuable for brain health.

Thank You, Pat Summitt!

We all owe a great debt of gratitude to Pat Summitt, the legendary coach of Tennessee's Lady Vols, a pioneer of women's athletics who has more victories on her scorecard than any other college coach in the game of basketball. Why? Not because of her coaching and athletic prowess, but because, at age 59 and at the peak of her career, she candidly announced to the world that she has been diagnosed with early onset Alzheimer's disease. No shame or embarrassment for the coach—and there shouldn't be for you or your loved one, either.

The healthy spouse might also find that friends stop visiting or calling because they don't know how to handle the situation. Be sure to find ways to keep your caregiver parent socially engaged. For example, your mom might not ask to go to dinner, shopping, or a movie with you, or even to come over to visit with the grandchildren. Likewise, she might not ask you to come over and watch your dad so she can visit with friends. You might need to prompt the request and create a support plan to make it possible.

Dementia is an illness that affects the entire family, and each member will respond differently. All of you can expect to feel new emotions, and that can be unsettling. Be patient with yourself and other family members as you face life with dementia and find your way to cope and care.

Dementia's Seeds of Discord

One of the more difficult concepts for some family members to grasp is that someone suffering from dementia is not deliberately acting difficult, nor does he or she mean every unkind thing said. Believing that dementia behavior is thoughtful and methodical will harvest seeds of discord throughout your caregiving.

Far too often—perhaps because of past history, unresolved conflicts, or old patterns of behavior—spouses or adult children react to the person with Alzheimer's disease or another form of dementia with a heightened sense of frustration. They "read into" the loved one's behavior because they are trying to make sense of it or because it might have touched a nerve. Mom or Dad's dementia isn't given the benefit of the doubt. And so those cutting words and that mean behavior give them cause for striking back, as if the aggravation had been intentionally inflicted.

People with dementia can sometimes appear to behave normally and act lucidly. I've had many caregivers laugh at this fact, telling me that those moments happen at the exact time their out-of-town sibling finally shows up to visit. As one caregiver described it, "I'd been telling my brother that Mom really couldn't be left alone any longer and that her dementia was getting worse. He showed up for a half-hour visit during one of her good days and called me a drama queen for overreacting."

Given the unpredictability of dementia and how it affects each person differently, some family members might find it hard to distinguish between when a loved one "really means" what is said or done and when the behavior is caused by the disease.

For example, a daughter might think that Mom "knows exactly what she is doing." If Mom says something hurtful, the daughter then interprets it as, "She's just out to get me." The daughter likely will respond in anger, an emotion that people with dementia easily sense through tone of voice and body language. In a matter of minutes, both people find themselves in the midst of a firestorm.

Another interpretation of dementia behavior is the conviction that whatever cruel or unkind statement Mom or Dad makes is "what Mom or Dad was thinking all along." In this scenario, a father who might have had a good relationship with his son starts blurting out damning statements, calling him "lazy" and accusing him of "just wanting all of my money." Now the son begins to doubt his treasured relationship with his father and wonders whether his dad thought this about him all along.

In both cases, if this is the premise you base your caregiving on—that upsetting words and acts are intentional and your parent has been masking these negative feelings all along—then you're headed for a great deal of heartache and dangerous levels of stress.

Tip

Meeting other people who are caring for a loved one with Alzheimer's disease and learning how they manage can give you priceless insights from those who are in your shoes. To find a support group anywhere in the country, go to www.alz.org, or give its 24-hour help line a call at 1-800-272-3900.

Dementia is a brain disease. Learn about it, talk to your doctor about it, and go to the Alzheimer's Association website to take a virtual tour of the brain and see what plaques and tangles are doing to parts of your loved one's brain. You'll see how the disease affects emotions, behavior, and motor function. The less you make your loved one's disease about you, the better.

Communicating with Someone Who Has Alzheimer's

Imagine how you feel when you're driving along and realize you're lost. At first, you might feel angry and frustrated that you can't figure out the directions. If you have a "backseat driver" who tries to help, you probably become all the more irritated. And if you've steered your way into parts unknown, you might feel threatened and scared, even though there really isn't anything to fear.

For people with Alzheimer's, the analogy is all too real. They feel frustrated, confused, and fearful in a world of strangers doing things to them or giving them "backseat" directions. They are in a constant state of being lost—nothing is familiar, not the room they live in, the furniture, the faces they see every day, their daily routines, or even their own family members. It's no wonder they exhibit anger or appear agitated.

So how do you talk to a person with Alzheimer's? How do you break past the fear, the anger, and the confusion? *Talking to Alzheimer's,* by Claudia J. Strauss, is full of savvy, simple advice. It would have been a great help to me during the year I cared at home for my grandmother-in-law who suffered from vascular dementia induced by a stroke. Here are some of Strauss's suggestions:

- **Calm down before you walk in to visit.** Your goal is to get yourself emotionally ready and to be at ease. Take some deep breaths, envision your favorite soothing place, or call up the feeling of someone rubbing your shoulders or back. Relax. Why? You'll want to convey a sense of peacefulness and readiness to enjoy your loved one when you enter the room. You're creating an oasis during your visit. You'll want to give off "good vibes," because that's what your loved one will pick up. It's best to enter the room with something like, "Hi, Dad, it's me, Linda, your daughter," so he won't have to guess or be embarrassed if he doesn't recognize you.

- **Understand that your loved one's reality has changed.** Setting Dad straight on facts and dates is not helpful. It will probably agitate him and remind him that he's losing his grasp of reality. If he thinks his mother is still alive or that his son is still small and needs to be picked up from school, simply show that you're listening instead of arguing (nod or say, "I hear what you're saying," or give a noncommittal "Uh huh," if you prefer not to lie).

- **Expect a lot of repetition.** Your loved one is struggling to remember the last conversation he had. He lives in the moment. Every time he asks a question, it is new to him, so you must act as if it is a new question to you, too. Answer in a tone of voice that is reassuring.

- **Ask questions that have a yes or no answer.** An open-ended question like "How is your day going, Mom?" is an exception, because it is in the here and now. Avoid questions that require retrieving information from memory. You don't want to place your family member on the spot so that she becomes embarrassed or angry with herself for not being able to remember.

Talking to Alzheimer's is full of examples of what to say and how to respond to a great number of common situations. In addition to Strauss's advice, here are other tips to help you communicate more effectively with your loved one:

- **Show interest in what your loved one is saying.** Maintain good eye contact, and don't interrupt or argue. Dad needs to know that you care about what he's telling you.

- **When holding a conversation, keep distractions to a minimum and use short sentences in plain words.** But don't use "baby talk" or talk in front of Dad as if he isn't in the room.

- **Use visual cues.** Point to what you are referring to (for example, the bathroom), use a picture board, or make gestures. If your dad is able to, ask him to show you what he means by doing the same. Or if he can't find the right word, try to guess the correct one.

- **Break down tasks or instructions into concrete, simple steps.** Don't overwhelm your dad with logic or quiz him. Remain patient while he gives a response; he needs the added time to process his answer.

- **Approach from the front when you're speaking.** Coming from behind might be startling.

- **Don't correct or argue with your loved one.** This will only frustrate both of you. Logically reasoning with someone who no longer has that capacity simply won't work.

Walk in My Shoes

Plenty of scholarly articles and books describe the stages of dementia and how people act and behave. But the book that helped me imagine and feel what it must be like to be diagnosed and live with Alzheimer's is a book of fiction by neuroscientist Lisa Genova, titled *Still Alice*.

Much of how you communicate with others is based on the feelings you convey to them. If your loved one can feel your warmth and respect and know that you like being together, the words you use are secondary.

When your loved one says things that are hurtful, take a deep breath and remind yourself that this isn't done on purpose. I know that it's far easier said than done, but don't take it personally. Mom or Dad is brain injured. Keep that one fact in the front of your mind; it will help you keep your emotions in check.

Establishing a New Normal

A spouse who is the primary caregiver for a person living with dementia is still a spouse. Letting go of the most significant relationship of a lifetime is ever so hard. But what makes it even tougher is letting go when the person you are "losing" isn't really lost. One of your parents might be caught up in a world filled with what Pauline Boss calls "ambiguous loss." For example, your mother has lost your dad in some ways, but in others, he is very much present. Your dad will have moments in which he is very aware and acts perfectly "normal," luring your mom into believing that he'll emerge from the fog.

But sadly, the man she's known and loved won't reappear. The hard work for your mother is to begin redefining her reality and her relationship with your father. She'll need some time while you and her close friends help her come to what experts call "a new normal." Your mother's task is to cherish what was, accept what is, and continue on with her life. This is also your task.

The Family Caregiver Alliance and Pauline Boss, author of *Ambiguous Loss,* offer a number of suggestions that might help your parent caregiver and you move toward a new kind of "normal." Here's what they suggest:

- **Spend time with friends and family in the "real" world.** Connect with people who are healthy and in the present, to give you a break from the roller-coaster "ins and outs" of reality when living with someone with dementia.

- **Identify your problem.** Understand that ambiguous loss is at the center of much of your stress, guilt, and anger. What you're losing is often vague, changing, and confusing. If you know that this is going on, you can better understand what you are reacting to and cope with it.

- **Understand that you no longer live in a world of either/or choices.** Making a choice that either you'll be your loved one's caregiver or not, or deciding that a perfect solution will emerge—either this or either that—just isn't realistic. Your life is about balancing two different ideas at the same time. It's about *both* instead of *either/or.* For example, you can be both sad that your loved one doesn't understand that the baby she's holding is her grandchild and yet happy while you soak up the joys of being a grandparent.

- **Revise family holidays and traditions.** This doesn't mean you should cancel family gatherings, nor does it mean you should isolate the individual with dementia and his or her caregiver. It means you should find ways to simplify holidays. For example, you might create a quieter space for Mom so she won't be overwhelmed by children running around or loud chatter among adults. Family members can sit with her while the caregiver visits and takes part in the celebration.

- **Find something new to hope for.** In addition to the physical incapacities that come with the disease, caring for someone with dementia is wearing both physically and mentally. Psychologists have found that hoping for something in the midst of adversity is a surefire antidepressant. Just the act of thinking about spending a little time on a hobby or developing a new one, meeting people in a support group and developing a new relationship, or looking forward to going out with friends provides the hope to go on and the reassurance that, despite all its hardships, life is worth living and good.

If you have a parent who is the primary caregiver, offer reassurance. For example, let Dad know that part of your job is to look out for him. He will likely have his own health issues that deserve attention, but under the stress and time constraints of caregiving, he might ignore them. Of course, the same advice applies to you, if you are the primary caregiver.

The Care Receiver's Values

Caregivers underestimate what a loved one with mild to moderate dementia values and wants from caregivers. That's the key finding of a recent study from Penn State University and the Benjamin Rose Institute on Aging.

This breakthrough study asked persons with dementia about *their* preferences and values. Most research is based on what caregivers think and feel in regard to their caregiving experience. So what can we learn from the study to better assist you in communicating with your loved one?

Because you'll make many decisions in the interest of your parent or spouse, it's helpful for them and you to know their preferences when you're acting on their behalf. Moreover, a person living with dementia *can* make some decisions, and you won't be in a position to respond to what Mom values if you don't know what she wants in the first place. If you're not in sync, you'll both become frustrated.

The researchers found that five core values are important to individuals with dementia:

- **Autonomy.** "I want to make everyday decisions, such as deciding what activities I'll do and at what time of day. Let me determine my routine and spend money on things I want."

- **Burden.** "I want to avoid becoming a physical, emotional, or financial burden to my family. And I don't want my caregiver to put his or her life on hold for me."

- **Control.** "I want to avoid family conflicts. Let me choose who I want to help with my care and exclude those I don't want caring for me. It's important to me that I'll be able to leave money to my family after my death."

- **Family.** "I want to have something to do that's meaningful for me and to be with family and friends. I want to be part of family gatherings and celebrations."

- **Safety.** "I want to be safe from crime and feel safe within my own home. It's important to me that I can be in touch with someone in case of an emergency."

On all these counts, caregivers didn't think that these values really mattered to their loved ones. Why the disconnect? According to Steven Zarit, professor and head of the Department of Human Development and Family Studies at Penn State and the study's leader, "[A] major reason for differences in these perceptions is that caregivers come to view people with dementia as unable to make their own decisions about daily life." In contrast, Zarit found that the people he talked to with mild and moderate dementia "remained capable of making decisions for themselves and could express their values in a clear and direct way."

As the disease progresses, of course, people with dementia can no longer make decisions in their best interest. But during mild and moderate stages, they can make choices that you can facilitate. It might take your loved one a little more time, and the results could even be a little messy, but it's worth reinforcing your parent's sense of self and independence.

During the early dementia stages, it's all the more urgent for you to learn what matters to your loved one, especially among the five core values we've reviewed. Once you've discussed this with your parent, you'll know how to truly act on his or her behalf when Mom or Dad can no longer express those wishes to you.

When I cared for my newborn son and his great-grandmother at the same time, I was tempted to simply dress Lena in the mornings. She was willing, but I knew it would be better for her if she made her own decisions on what dress and sweater she would wear and how she would do her hair for the day. Each decision would give her brain a workout, to stave off the quick deterioration of her vascular dementia. But some days, I was simply too exhausted or in too much of a hurry responding to a crying infant in the other room. I learned to forgive myself and start fresh the next day, with new decisions for Grandma to make—and even some involving her great-grandson.

For example, you could ask your mom how much she enjoys attending family get-togethers. If she enjoys this, ask her how you can make it comfortable for her. Does she like being part of the festivities, with everyone coming and going? Is she okay with children running around, or would she rather be in a side room calmly visiting with a few people at a time? Because some people with dementia can become easily agitated or anxious, caregivers might assume that the parent wouldn't be interested in attending a family event. Yet with some sensitive planning and a willing heart, it can be done.

Essential Takeaways

- If your parent is diagnosed with dementia, plan on making this a family affair. Everyone is affected, and each of you will respond and adjust in your own way.
- Despite the dementia, your loved one cares about the future, doesn't want to be a burden, wants to make decisions about his or her care, and doesn't like conflict.
- If you believe your loved one is intentionally saying things to hurt you or has secretly felt this way about you all along, you're headed for a great deal of stress and heartache.
- You *can* communicate with your loved one. Take the time to learn how, listen, be patient, and soak in the joy of connecting.

Resource Directory

There are a ton of resources available to assist caregivers. You'll find them on the internet and among organizations; many of them have chapters in your community. It can be overwhelming to search and sort through lists of services, so here are over 60 resources with short descriptions on what they offer and how to contact them, giving you quick access to the services you need. This entire directory is available at www. lindarhodescaregiving.com, where all the websites are hyperlinked for your convenience.

Health and Medicine

Alcoholics Anonymous (AA)
Phone: 212-870-3400
Website: www.alcoholics-anonymous.org

Check your phone book first for a local chapter. AA offers support to alcoholics and their families. Click on "Is There an Alcoholic in Your Life?" to help answer questions about family members and loved ones.

Alzheimer's Association
Phone: 1-800-272-3900
Website: www.alz.org

This is an excellent organization that offers a wide range of information and support services. The website provides a caregiver's guide, an "Ask the Expert" online feature, medical information, videos, and a locator to find your local Alzheimer's chapter.

Alzheimer's Disease Education and Referral Center
Phone: 1-800-438-4380
Website: www.nia.nih.gov/alzheimers

This site provides the latest information on new treatments. You can track current clinical trials and find out how to connect to 20 national Alzheimer's disease centers throughout the country. The site also keeps you posted on results of the most recent research studies.

American Diabetes Association
Phone: 1-800-342-2383
Website: www.diabetes.org

The association's website is extensive, giving you the latest in research, general information, nutrition, news, lifestyle tips, and links to other great sources. On this site, you can also find local chapters near you.

American Heart Association
Phone: 1-800-242-8721
Website: www.americanheart.org

This group provides research, information, and education about the heart. Click on an extensive site map to see what's available. Included are warning signs of heart attacks and stroke, separate sections on women, patient information, and links to other sites.

The American Lung Association
Phone: 1-800-586-4872
Website: www.lungusa.org

Contact a local chapter by entering your zip code on the website. Search the site for information on all lung topics, such as asbestos, air quality, tobacco, and tuberculosis. View and download free pamphlets.

Arthritis Foundation
Phone: 1-800-283-7800
Website: www.arthritis.org

This foundation offers very good consumer health information on the prevention and treatment of arthritis. It provides information and referral services to a local chapter, support groups, and classes. The website also has a product store and a section on advocacy.

Healthfinder
Website: www.healthfinder.gov

This is a gateway site to consumer health and human services information from the U.S. Department of Health and Human Services. It's a great site that's easy to use, with links to agencies and databases and a directory of services.

Hearing Loss Association of America
Phone: 301-657-2248
Website: www.hearingloss.org

This nonprofit educational organization offers assistance and resources for people with hearing loss and helps families learn to adjust to living with an affected member. Resources are available on the website, in *Hearing Loss Magazine,* and through webinars.

Lighthouse International
Phone: 1-800-829-0500
Website: www.lighthouse.org

This national center provides valuable information for those with vision problems, including simulations of what someone with macular degeneration and other age-related eye disorders actually see. It features a terrific online catalog of devices that can make life easier and improve vision. It also offers a locator for finding low-vision clinics and practitioners that assess eye health and recommend adaptive strategies, medications, and treatment.

MEDLINEplus
Website: www.medlineplus.gov

This is the site for the National Library of Medicine and National Institutes of Health. If you want to bookmark just one site for your medical information, this is it. It's a terrific resource for all kinds of medical information linking you to other resources. Click on the drug information site to review reports on thousands of prescription and over-the-counter drugs.

Mental Health America (formerly National Mental Health Association)
Phone: 1-800-969-6642
Website: www.mentalhealthamerica.net

This organization has 240 local affiliates dedicated to improving mental health and conquering mental illnesses. The website has an information center to help you find affiliates and obtain publications. Click on "Confidential depression-screening test" to gauge your (or a loved one's) depression.

National Association for Continence
Phone: 1-800-252-3337
Website: www.nafc.org

This site provides public education and advocacy about causes, prevention, diagnosis, treatment, and management alternatives for incontinence.

National Coalition for Cancer Survivorship
Phone: 1-877-622-7937
Website: www.canceradvocacy.org

This is a patient-led organization for patients with cancer and their families. The website includes a "Cancer Resources" section with a "Cancer Survival Toolbox" series, a section to listen to audiotapes, and a place to view transcripts.

National Council on Alcohol and Drug Dependence
Phone: 212-269-7797; 1-800-622-2255 for affiliate referral
Website: www.ncadd.org

This is a nationwide, voluntary organization that deals with alcoholism and other drug addictions. It provides education and information, along with advocacy efforts. You can get assistance by calling the 800-number or entering your zip code to identify the closest NCADD affiliate.

National Eye Institute
Phone: 301-496-5248
Website: www.nei.nih.gov

This institute specializes in vision, research, and information for professionals, the public, media, and educators. The website has a search function, eye charts, videos, online publications, and a great site map.

National Health Information Center
Phone: 1-800-336-4797
Website: www.health.gov/NHIC/

This is a multipurpose website designed to help the general public and professionals find health information. It includes a listing of health-related organizations (with links) and a list of toll-free numbers for assistance.

National Heart, Lung and Blood Institute
Phone: 301-592-8573
Website: www.nhlbi.nih.gov

Here you can find excellent information on diseases of the heart, lung, and blood. You can also learn about the latest results of studies, news, and clinical trials.

National Institute of Diabetes, Digestive and Kidney Diseases
Phone: 301-496-3583
Website: www.niddk.nih.gov

This institute offers a wealth of information on diabetes, digestive diseases, and kidney diseases. It gives you the latest research results, includes a clinical trial finder, presents understandable health information, and offers links to other helpful sites on preventing and controlling these diseases.

National Institute of Mental Health
Phone: 1-866-615-6464
Website: www.nimh.nih.gov

Get the latest information on symptoms research, diagnosis, and treatment of mental illness. Call for brochures, fact sheets, and other materials.

National Institute of Neurological Disorders and Stroke
Phone: 1-800-352-9424
Website: www.ninds.nih.gov

The institute offers a top-notch website that describes brain attacks and offers prevention strategies. It also offers information on other brain disorders, such as Parkinson's, Alzheimer's, and epilepsy. You can also get referrals to local clinical research centers.

National Institute on Aging

Phone: 301-496-1752
Website: www.nih.gov/nia/

This website includes a resource directory, with links to other aging-related sites, as well as a list of "Age Pages" on various topics related to aging that are available to the public. You can read the "Age Pages" online.

National Institutes of Health

Phone: 301-496-4000
Website: www.nih.gov

This federal agency houses a wide range of health institutes cited in this appendix. By visiting this gateway site, you can link to other institutes, find clinical trials for most diseases throughout the country, and review the data on prescription and over-the-counter drugs.

National Osteoporosis Foundation

Phone: 1-800-231-4222
Website: www.nof.org

The website of this consumer- and patient-focused organization has a lot of information on preventing osteoporosis and broken bones and promoting strong bones throughout all stages of life. Get the latest news, advocacy efforts, prevention tips, awareness kits, brochures, videos (for free and for sale), and information about talking to your doctor about your bone health. Since there is no osteoporosis specialty among doctors, the Find a Healthcare Professional and Newly Diagnosed buttons at the top of the home page are particularly helpful.

National Sleep Foundation

Phone: 202-347-3471
Website: www.sleepfoundation.org

Here you'll find great information on sleep disorders and treatment. You can also find sleep clinic details on the website.

National Stroke Association
Phone: 1-800-787-6537
Website: www.stroke.org

The association offers a wide range of information on strokes. It makes referrals to medical experts, rehab centers, and support groups. The website offers good links to other related sites.

Paralyzed Veterans of America
Phone: 1-800-424-8200
Website: www.pva.org

This veteran's service organization focuses on special needs of veterans with spinal cord dysfunction. Issues include health care, research, education, benefits, civil rights, and opportunities for paralyzed veterans.

Parkinson's Resource Organization
Phone: 1-877-775-4111
Website: www.parkinsonsresource.org

This organization, established in 1990, provides emotional and educational support through an interactive website, monthly newsletters, support groups, and one-on-one coaching.

Death and Dying

Aging with Dignity
Phone: 850-681-2010 or 1-888-594-7437
Website: www.agingwithdignity.org

This is a privately funded nonprofit organization that places special emphasis on improving care for the elderly at the end of their lives. Five Wishes is an easy-to-understand living will, or advance directive, for all ages. Click on "Five Wishes" on the website for a preview.

American Hospice Foundation
Phone: 202-223-0204 or 1-800-347-1413
Website: www.americanhospice.org

This organization provides you with helpful information on hospice care. Referrals to a hospice near your parent, counseling resources, and support programs are available on its website.

Growth House, Inc.
Website: www.growthhouse.org

This group is billed as the "internet's leading online community for end of life care." It is a gateway site to resources for life-threatening illnesses and end-of-life care. You get great information and group support through chat rooms.

National Hospice and Palliative Care Organization
Phone: 1-800-658-8898
Website: www.caringinfo.org

This consumer website offers information on hospice and palliative care, advance care planning, caring for others, and more.

The National Hospice and Palliative Care Organization with the American Bar Association wrote a practical, easy, how-to guide that helps families navigate the essential steps of getting their affairs in order. The seven steps show you how to pay for health care, manage health and personal decisions, administer money and property, plan for the care of dependents, know your rights as an employee, be aware of your rights as a patient, and complete various legal documents.

You can access the "Legal Guide for the Seriously Ill: Seven Key Steps to Get Your Affairs" by going to www.lindarhodescaregiving.org and viewing "Caregiver Tips."

Government Agencies and Services

Access America for Seniors
Website: www.seniors.gov
Phone: 1-800-FED-INFO (1-800-333-4636)

This is a government-wide initiative to deliver electronic services from government agencies and organizations to seniors. It's a one-stop website for anyone who wants information on senior issues, from A to Z. It links to your state's Department of Aging site.

Administration on Aging
Website: www.aoa.gov

This is the federal agency that acts as the hub for all government aging services and provides the network of state and area agencies on aging. The website is chock full of information and links to other related government sites.

Department of Veterans Affairs
Phone: 1-800-827-1000
Website: www.va.gov

This federal agency operates all of veteran's services. The website is excellent and will save you a great deal of time. You can determine your parents' benefits, see who qualifies for what, and learn how to apply. Contact information is provided, and you can download and print application forms.

The Veterans Administration also offers a VA Caregiver Support program, at www.caregiver.va.gov, or call the Support Line at 1-855-260-3274. All eligible veterans may qualify for a range of long-term care services, including skilled nursing, home health care, adult day center services, vehicle modifications, respite care, and more.

Eldercare Locator
Phone: 1-800-677-1116
Website: www.eldercare.gov

This service is offered by the federal Administration on Aging (AOA). If you call and describe your problem, someone will direct you to local and regional agencies for senior services and to your local Area Agency on Aging. You can also get this information by visiting the website.

Housing and Urban Development (HUD)
Phone: 1-888-569-4287
Website: www.hud.gov

This federal agency runs low-income housing for seniors. Visit its website to find out whether your parent qualifies for federal congregate housing and other housing services. The site includes information on resources to help older persons stay at home; how to find an apartment or service-supported house; and how to combat discrimination, fraud, and reverse mortgage scams. Click on "Topic Areas" and "Information for Senior Citizens."

Medicare Hotline
Phone: 1-800-MEDICARE (1-800-633-4227)
Website: www.medicare.gov

Call the Medicare Hotline to inquire about plans and what HMOs offer service in your area, to get brochures mailed to you, or to complain about problems or report fraud. At the website, you can type in "Nursing Home Compare" and get the latest inspection reports on every nursing home in the country.

Social Security Administration (SSA)
Phone: 1-800-772-1213
Website: www.ssa.gov

The SSA is the federal agency that runs Social Security retirement, survivors' benefits, disability insurance, and SSI (Supplemental Security Income). The website is an award-winning government site, is easy to use, and answers most of your questions. It offers a directory of local offices.

Caregiving Resources

Caring Bridge
Phone: 651-789-2300
Website: www.caringbridge.org

Caring Bridge provides free, personal and private websites that connect people going through a significant health challenge among family and friends. The websites are easy to create and use, but if you have a question, you can call for help in walking through the process. Family members post photos and updates on their loved one's health, and visitors leave messages of hope and support in the guestbook. This saves time and energy for caregivers while keeping family and friends in the loop.

Family Caregiver Alliance
Phone: 1-800-445-8106
Website: www.caregiver.org

This is the website for the National Center on Caregiving. It is an information hub for programs, services, fact sheets, policy and research papers, and consumer articles on a wide range of topics facing family caregivers. It includes features blogs, discussion groups, and a Family Care Navigator, which is a listing of services by state.

Family Caregiving 101
Website: www.familycaregiving101.org

The National Alliance for Caregiving and the National Family Caregivers Association teamed up to provide families the basic tools and information they need to navigate health care, understand the stages of caregiving, and track down resources.

National Adult Day Services Association
Website: www.nadsa.org

Mostly a website for association members, this site has a consumer section that offers a Site Visit Check List, fact sheet on adult day services, and a locator to find a center near you.

National Association of Professional Geriatric Care Managers
Phone: 520-881-8008
Website: www.caremanager.org

This is an association of member geriatric professionals that emphasizes advocacy, education, and standards of care for the elderly.

National Family Caregivers Association
Phone: 1-800-896-3650
Website: www.nfcacares.org

This is a national charitable organization for caregivers. It provides assistance in the areas of information and education, support and validation, and public awareness and advocacy. Its website is comprehensive.

General Resources

AAA Foundation for Traffic Safety
Phone: 1-800-305-7233
Website: www.aaafoundation.org

This is a nonprofit research organization focused on driver education, safety, and prevention. You can order free brochures on driving and the older driver, or buy videotapes about older drivers and safety issues. Several written driving tests for the older driver can help families deal with difficult issues.

Abledata Assistive Technology
Phone: 1-800-227-0216
Website: www.abledata.com

This organization catalogs assistive technology. Product information and price ranges are included on the website. The National Institute on Disability and Rehabilitation Research of the Department of Education funds the site but does not endorse any of the products.

Alliance for Retired Americans
Phone: 202-607-5399
Website: www.retiredamericans.org

Created in the 2001 reorganization of the National Council of Senior Citizens (NCSC), the Alliance works to unite seniors in advocating for legislation and policies that respond to their interests at the national, state, and local levels.

American Association of Retired Persons (AARP)
Phone: 1-800-424-3410
Website: www.aarp.org

The website of this educational and action organization for those 50 and older is excellent. To find information on caring for an aging parent, type "caregiver" into the search box. AARP members can take advantage of the AARP Legal Services Network (www.aarp.org/lsn), a free first consultation with a lawyer.

Center for Medicare Advocacy
Phone: 1-860-456-7790
Website: www.medicareadvocacy.org

This is a private, nonprofit foundation that focuses on health-care rights, especially the needs of Medicare beneficiaries. The website has links to other sites that emphasize Medicare.

Commission on Legal Problems of the Elderly
Phone: 202-662-8690
Website: www.abanet.org/elderly

The commission focuses on improving legal services for the elderly, with involvement of the private bar. It deals with elderly legal issues that surround HMOs, elder abuse, guardianship, and others. You can download an advance directive. (The commission is not active in all states.)

Leading Age (formerly American Association of Homes and Services for the Aging)
Phone: 202-783-2242
Website: www.leadingage.org

This group represents 5,000 not-for-profit facilities that care for the aging and those in assisted living facilities. Click on the section designated "Looking for Information on Aging Services." Search by city, state, zip code, and type of facility or service to find a not-for-profit nursing home, assisted living facility, or community-based service.

Meals on Wheels Association of America
Phone: 703-548-5558
Website: www.mowaa.org

Track down the number of the local Meals on Wheels program in your area to have meals delivered to your parent's home or to volunteer. Or check your local phone book for Meals on Wheels.

Medicare Rights Center
Phone: 1-800-333-4114
Website: www.medicarerights.org

This national, nonprofit organization advocates for affordable health care for older adults and those with disabilities. You'll find plenty of easy-to-understand information on Medicare, a Medicare Interactive tool to answer your questions, and information to stay up-to-date on Medicare legislation. The site and helpline are also available in Spanish.

National Academy of Elder Law Attorneys, Inc.
Website: www.naela.org

This nonprofit association provides information, education, networking, and assistance to those who deal with the specialized issues of legal services to the elderly and disabled. The website also has a function that helps you find elder law attorneys in your area.

National Association for Home Care and Hospice
Phone: 202-547-7424
Website: www.nahc.org

This nonprofit group has an excellent website on home health care so you can learn about all the different services and therapies available under home care. The site offers a home care and hospice locator, as well as a guide on choosing a home care provider.

National Caucus and Center on Black Aged
Phone: 202-637-8400
Website: www.ncba-aged.org

The center's mission is to enhance the quality of life among aging African Americans. It is not a service provider; however, it addresses programs in employment, health care, housing options, and long-term care.

National Center for Home Equity Conversion
Phone: 1-800-218-1415
Website: www.reverse.org

This website is devoted to the consumer. Click "Calculator" to get an instant estimate of your home equity. Review the sources in your state for reverse equity home mortgages. Learn all you could possibly want to know about reverse mortgages before you make any decisions.

National Consumers League
Phone: 202-835-3323
Website: www.nclnet.org

This is a private, nonprofit group advertised as the oldest consumer's group in the United States. It represents consumers on all workplace and market-place issues. One click gives you access to information on telemarketing, internet fraud, and drug interactions.

National Council on the Aging
Phone: 202-479-1200
Website: www.ncoa.org

This organization of agencies and professionals states that its mission is to "help community organizations enhance the lives of older adults." Click on "Aging Issues" and then on "Caregiving" for information.

National Shared Housing Resource Center
Website: www.nationalsharedhousing.org

This is a nonprofit national clearinghouse for information on shared housing. On the website, click on "Directory" and then choose a state to get the name, address, and phone number of a program, as well as a thumbnail description.

The National Women's Health Information Center
Office of Women's Health, DHHS
Phone: 1-800-994-9662
Website: www.4women.gov

This website focuses on women's issues. Use the search box by entering "aging," "caregiver," or "elder care" for a multitude of excellent direct links. Resource information is available on Alzheimer's, ways to empower caregivers and working women, and elder care.

Visiting Nurse Associations (VNA) of America
Phone: 1-800-426-2547
Website: www.vnaa.org

More than 500 VNAs operate throughout the country, providing skilled nursing, hospice, home health aides, homemakers, nutrition advice, and personal assistance. Find a VNA near you and ask if your parent is eligible for home health care.

Videos

If you'd like to see how to give someone with Alzheimer's a bath without a huge argument, how to transfer a loved one in and out of bed or a chair without injuring your back, and better understand how dementia affects the brain, among many other caregiving videos, you can visit two different websites: www.learningcenter.pahomecare.org (sponsored by the Pennsylvania Homecare Association) and www.videocaregiving.org (offered by Terra Nova Films). All the videos are free to view. Also visit my website for "Caregiver Minutes" at www.lindarhodescaregiving.com.

Caregiver Forms

Effective caregiving calls for being organized and knowing how to break down problems to find workable solutions. The Master Contact List provides a simple tool to identify all those involved in your parent's care (for example, doctors, home health providers, hired caregivers, family members, and service providers). The Caregiving Task Assessment Worksheet helps you determine what your loved one needs, and the Caregiving Resource Assessment Worksheet can be used to identify who or what can address each care need (refer back to Chapter 3 for filled-out examples).

You can access these forms, fill them out, download them, and print them at www.lindarhodescaregiving. com.

Master Contact List

LindaRhodes
caregiving

For (Name of Care Receiver): _____

Name of Primary Caregiver: _____

Caregiver Phone Numbers: (Home): _____ (Office): _____ (Cell): _____

Type of Contact (e.g. doctor, nurse, pharmacy, adult day care center, clinic)	Name of Contact (Person's name that you usually speak to)	Phone Number	Notes

LindaRhodes
caregiving™

Part 1: Adult Daily Living Tasks	Level of Help Needed		
Task/Activity Description	None	Some	A Lot
1. Bathing:			
Sponge bath	___	___	___
Shower	___	___	___
Full bath	___	___	___
2. Dressing (putting on clothes)			
3. Grooming (hair, shave, teeth)			
4. Assist with walking:			
Needs a person to asisst	___	___	___
Uses walker	___	___	___
Uses cane	___	___	___
Uses wheelchair	___	___	___
5. Getting in and out of chair/bed			
6. Assist with going to the toilet			
7. Incontinence care (adult briefs, catheter)			
8. Meal preparation:			
Makes own meal	___	___	___
Arrange food on plate/cut food	___	___	___
Place food in mouth	___	___	___
9. Medication Reminding (hand them pills)			
10. Pill Organizing (sort pills/place in dispenser)			
11. How much do they interact with others?			

Part 2: Instrumental Adult Daily Living Tasks	Level of Help Needed		
Task/Activity Description	None	Some	A Lot
1. Shopping (e.g. groceries, clothes)			
2. Light houskeeping			
3. Do laundry			
4. Handle the mail			
5. Schedule and go to doctor appointments			
6. Drive			
7. Manage Money (e.g. pay bills, checking acct)			
8. Household chores (garbage, repairs)			
9. Handle health insurance matters (Medicare)			
10. Pill Organizing (sort pills/place in dispenser)			

LindaRhodes
caregiving

Caregiver Resource Assessment Worksheet

Task/Activity Description	Time Required Hours x per Week/Month	Resource Person(s)	Cost per Week/Month

Medical Forms

Providing physicians and health-care providers with up-to-date medical information is vital to your loved one's health and safety. It can literally be a lifesaver. The Medical Biography form can save you time listing health conditions for every new specialist your loved one sees. You can use the Med Minder form to list the medications your mom or dad is taking; you can then provide copies of this at every physician office visit. The My Medical Data form can be shared with paramedics so they'll easily and quickly know your loved one's health conditions, medications, allergies, and emergency contacts.

You can access these forms, fill them out, download them, and print them at www.lindarhodescaregiving. com.

Medical Biography

LindaRhodes
caregiving

Name	DOB	Date	Conditions (e.g. diabetes, heart)

Conditions (continued)

Allergies

List surgery or procedure	Physician	Hospital/Clinic	Date	Complications?
1.				
For:				
2.				
For:				
3.				
For:				
4.				
For:				
5.				
For:				
6.				
For:				

FAMILY HISTORY SNAPSHOT (List any diseases e.g. cancer, diabetes, high blood pressure of parents and siblings)

Conditions of Mother (Living: Yes or No / Age of Death)	Conditions of Father (Living: Yes or No / Age of Death)	Conditions of Siblings	Brother	Sister

Med Minder

LindaRhodes
caregiving

Name	DOB	Date	Conditions (e.g. diabetes, heart)

Conditions (continued)

Allergies

PRESCRIPTION DRUGS   Physician   (check one)   Enter how many pills for each time of the day:

Drug Name (e.g. Plavix) For: blood thinner	Generic	Brand	Dose	AM	Lunch	Dinner	Bedtime
1. For:							
2. For:							
3. For:							
4. For:							
5. For:							
6. For:							

OVER THE COUNTER DRUGS

Enter how many pills for each tie of the day:

Drug Name	Dose	AM	Lunch	Dinner	Bedtime

My Medical Data
LindaRhodes
caregiving™

Name _____

Date of Birth _____

Address _____

I AM ALLERGIC TO:

MEDICATIONS THAT I TAKE:

Drug Name	Dose	Drug Name	Dose

MY MEDICAL CONDITIONS: (such as I wear a pacemaker, or I am a diabetic)

MY FAMILY MEMBERS TO CONTACT:

Name & Relationship (son, spouse, daughter)	Phone Numbers (home, office, cell)

MY PRIMARY PHYSICIAN:

Name: _____ **Phone:** _____

Hospital of Choice: _____

Index

D

E

F

GCM. *See* geriatric care manager
gender bias, 223
generational gap, 205, 211
 baby boomers, 207-209
 common ground, 217
 denial, 214
 description of generations, 206
 Greatest Generation, 206-207, 213
 identity, 218
 negligent health-care choices, 214
 parent card, 216
 self-neglect, 214
 Silent Generation, 206
 view of doctors, 211
geriatric assessments, 19
geriatric care manager (GCM), 85-87,
 246, 284
geriatric emergency rooms, 183
"good child" motivator, 30
Greatest Generation, 24, 206, 211, 213
group homes, 119
guardianship, 136
guilt, 70-71

HCBS. *See* Home and Community-
 Based Services
HDL. *See* high-density lipoprotein
Health Insurance Portability and
 Accountability Act (HIPAA),
 154-156
health maintenance organization
 (HMO), 159
Health Proponent, 171

health records, 152-154
heart attacks, 7-8
hemorrhagic stroke, 10
hereditary units, 4
high blood pressure, 7
high-density lipoprotein (HDL), 8
high-touch human services, 110
HIPAA. *See* Health Insurance Portability and Accountability Act
HMO. *See* health maintenance organization
Home and Community-Based Services (HCBS), 101
home health care, 93-94, 165
hormonal substances, decline, 4
hormones, stress and, 64
hospice care, 198-199
hospitalized parent, 173
 bottom line, 176
 Center for Medicare Advocacy, 176
 choice of hospital, 173
 consumer groups, 176
 early discharge, 181-182
 economic choices of hospitals, 174
 emergency rooms, 183
 hospitalist, 177-178
 informed decisions, 185
 inpatient status, 175
 medical errors, 179
 primary care doctor, questions for,
 178
 survey, 174
HUD. *See* U.S. Department of
 Housing and Urban Development
human growth factors, 4

N–O

P

Q–R

S